MARK DENISON

LIFE
RECOVERY
PLAN

A 52-WEEK
GUIDE
TO KEEP
YOUR
RECOVERY
ON TRACK

*Because it's not enough to BECOME sexually sober
unless you STAY sexually sober.*

Life Recovery Plan: A 52-Week Guide to Keep Your Recovery on Track
Mark Denison D.Min.

ISBN: 978-1-7333130-5-6
Library of Congress Control Number: 2020907843

Cover design by Laurie Barboza - Design Stash Books
(DesignStashBooks@gmail.com)

Printed in the United States of America
2020 -- First Edition

Published by Austin Brothers Publishing

Fort Worth, Texas

DEDICATION

I dedicate this book to the men and women for whom finding recovery is not enough. They want to walk in recovery for the rest of their lives.

Table of Contents

INTRODUCTION

Two monumental tasks face every man and woman who suffers from a sexual addiction. He or she must (a) get sober, and then (b) stay sober. This book addresses the latter. As such, we seek to fill the gaping hole in the recovery plan of millions of addicts. They have jumped into the recovery process with desperation and intentionality. They have committed to any number of strategies: 12-Step groups, therapy, treatment centers, 90 meetings in 90 days, and more. Many have completed the 12 Steps or some other recovery process.

They may think they have graduated, but there is no graduation ceremony for the porn or sex addict. And there's a reason for that. Recovery is less about what you know than it is about what you do. So what are the options for continued care for the person who has already achieved a solid period of sobriety?

Every program has its limitations. For the 12-Step person, there is no 13th Step. For the person in therapy, his trauma and abuse issues have been addressed and treatment has been completed. For the person who has been "healed," there are still intrusive thoughts, painful memories, periods of isolation, and unforeseen challenges that must be countered.

That's where we come in. My own search for continued recovery material that was designed, not to help me find recovery, but to maintain it, left me frustrated and wanting. That was the genesis of this project. **Life Recovery Plan** is not for the person who is new to recovery. It is not for the man or woman seeking a diploma that signifies graduation. Rather, this workbook is designed for the millions of recovering addicts whose focus has shifted from finding recovery to keeping it.

Since I wrote **A 90-Day Recovery Guide for Sex Addicts**, I have known that something more was needed for the men who have completed this course. As I have led them through personal exercises, devotions, and intense recovery work, I have been amazed at the success of this program. But eventually, the 90 days run out.

Then what?

Recovery is for life, and this workbook is for life, as well. After extensive research and years of preparation, I have concluded two things: (a) recovery is for life, and (b) there are very specific themes/topics that address continued recovery more successfully than others. I have narrowed the scope of a lifetime of recovery to 52 of these themes; each must be mastered. And unlike the 12-Steps or my 90-Day Recovery Plan, you can jump into this process at any point. Each week's work stands alone, and there is no hierarchy or order to them.

This book consists of 52 weeks of work, which can—and should—be repeated from year to year. While you will benefit from reading straight through the book, there is a more intentional plan that will provide you with practical tools that will help secure a lifetime of recovery. This is how you should use this workbook:

1. Do the daily readings. There are seven readings that support each week's focus. The devotions will fuel your recovery and complement your written assignments.
2. Complete the weekly exercises. With each theme or topic, there is a creative exercise to complete. Take these seriously, and do not rush them.
3. Join a group. Our ministry, *There's Still Hope*, is providing groups, both in person and electronically, which I lead myself. Each group works through the workbook. You can jump in anytime, regardless of which week (topic) the group is on at the time.

While this *Life Recovery Plan* will be the missing piece of your lifetime of recovery, our ministry offers much more. Following are some of our other resources. Contact us for more information.

1. 90-Day Recovery Plan: I take men through this jump-start to their recovery, based on my book, *A 90-Day Recovery Guide*. The process includes daily readings, daily exercises, and a weekly coaching call which I lead myself.
2. Partner Recovery Group: My wife, Beth, leads online groups for women who are married to sex addicts. This 12-week process is based on her book, *12-Week Partner Recovery Workbook*.
3. Recovery Minute: This is my daily devotion, which I send by email to men and women all over the world. To sign up, visit our website at TheresStillHope.org.
4. Couples Intensive: Beth and I provide a one-day recovery intensive that features the latest in recovery resources for married couples.
5. Coaching for wives: Beth works with women, one-on-one, in navigating their own recovery.
6. Public speaking: Beth and I love to speak at churches, conferences, and schools.

7. Written resources: Our books include **Porn in the Pew, Porn-Free in 40 Days, A 90-Day Recovery Guide, 365 Days to Sexual Integrity,** and **Jesus & the 12 Steps**.

Week 1
Acceptance

"Let us not seek the Republican answer or the Democratic answer, but the right answer. Let us not seek to fix the blame for the past. Let us accept our own responsibility for the future."

\- John F. Kennedy

THIS WEEK'S EXERCISE
10 Signs You Are an Addict

Acceptance is where healing begins. Step 1 for Sexaholics Anonymous states it clearly: "We admitted that we were powerless over lust—that our lives had become unmanageable." Still, some want a more clinical definition of addiction before they admit to a real problem.

For that we turn to Dr. Adrian Hickmon, founder of Capstone Treatment Center. Hickmon holds a Ph.D. in Marriage and Family Therapy from Virginia Tech and an MA in Substance Abuse Counseling from Northeast Louisiana University. He is also a Licensed Professional Counselor, a Marriage and Family Therapist, and Certified Sex Addiction Therapist, with over 25,000 hours of actual therapy experience.

In other words, Dr. Hickmon knows what he's talking about.

Hickmon lists ten signs of addiction. Check the ones which describe you.

Criteria of Sexual Addiction

1. **Loss of control:** clear behavior in which you do more than you intend or want

2. **Compulsive behavior:** a pattern of out of control behavior over time

3. **Efforts to stop:** repeated specific attempts to stop the behavior which have failed

4. **Loss of time:** significant amounts of time lost doing and/or recovering from the behavior

5. **Preoccupation:** obsessing about or because of the behavior

6. **Inability to fulfill obligations:** the behavior interferes with work, school, family, and friends

7. **Continuation despite negative consequences**: failure to stop the behavior even though you have problems because of it (social, legal, financial, physical)

8. **Escalation**: need to make behavior more intense, more frequent, or more risky

9. **Losses**: losing, limiting, or sacrificing valued parts of life such as hobbies, family relationships, and work

10. **Withdrawal**: stopping behavior causes considerable distress, anxiety, restlessness, irritability, or physical discomfort

How many of these did you check? What does this mean? Dr. Hickmon says that if you checked three or more of the above, then you are likely an addict. If you checked more than five, there is really no doubt about it.

Day 1
Lesson from Jimmy Connors

We cannot get well until we get real. We must admit we have a problem. That is the first step of the 12 steps and the foundation of all recovery.

Say it with me: "I have a problem."

I read an anonymous quote that I have committed to memory. "I would rather go through life sober, believing that I am an alcoholic, than go through life drunk, trying to convince myself that I am not."

You will never know how good things can be until you admit how bad things already are. Your addiction, relapse, and failures can become the launching pad of your success.

Legendary tennis player Jimmy Connors said, "Treat relapse not as a failure, but as a challenge."

Admit your problem to God. Then get ready for the ride of your life. "The God of all grace, who called you to his eternal glory in Christ, after you have suffered a little while, will himself restore you and make you strong, firm, and steadfast" (1 Peter 5:10).

You can have a better future, but first, you must quit trying to have a better past. The sooner you accept your struggle, the quicker you can overcome it.

Day 2
The $125,000 Penny

Michael Tremonti is a coin collector. Don't misunderstand. Michael isn't into paying big bucks for small coins. He buys common coins by the roll. For example, in October of 2018, Michael bought a roll of 1969 pennies. He paid about $10. So imagine his surprise when he sorted through the coins and found a rare 1969-S penny with a major flaw. Due to an error at the San Francisco mint, the date was fuzzy. It's what is known in the world of numismatics as a "double dye." The coin was authenticated by expert Ken Potter and valued at $125,000.

It is estimated that this coin had been possessed by dozens of bankers and hundreds of other citizens. To them it was worth one cent. Only in the hands of a true collector did the penny realize its full value. And while Michael's penny is in excellent condition, even a well-worn 1969-S double dye cent is worth $44,000. Compare that to a pristine, brilliantly uncirculated unflawed 1969-S penny, worth two cups of coffee at Starbucks.

Every recovering addict is flawed. We are worn, scarred, and blemished. But like the 1969-S penny, in the hands of the One who knows our real value, we are priceless.

The Bible praises the life of Moses. "It was by faith that Moses left the land of Egypt. He kept his eyes on the one who is invisible" (Hebrews 11:27).

Moses remains a hero to the Jews. He was without flaw—unless you count his self-doubt, impulsive behavior, and the day he murdered a total stranger in cold blood.

Michael Tremonti's penny is of great value, not because of its condition, but because of its owner. The same was true for Moses. And the same is true for you. You aren't of great value *despite* your flaws, but *because* of them.

Day 3
Disappointment

Disappointment. Trauma. Abuse. Isolation.

These are at the root of most personal struggles. Deep-seated disappointment in childhood produces great challenges in adulthood.

One of America's foremost experts on human sexuality, Dr. Jay Stringer, released his widely acclaimed book, *Unwanted: How Sexual Brokenness Reveals Our Way to Healing*, in 2018. He writes, "The real problem behind unwanted sexual behavior is an inability to deal with anxiety and disappointment."

If this sounds like you, I offer two suggestions.

First, define your value by the price God has put on your head. "While we were still sinners, Christ died for us" (Romans 5:8).

Second, know that no matter what, God is still there. He promises, "I will not forget you" (Isaiah 49:15).

Disappointment—it hurts, wounds, and inflicts emotional pain that can last a lifetime. But it doesn't have to be that way. We have a God who brings healing where there was pain and shines light where there s darkness.

Day 4
Off the Rails

Here's a powerful thought for this pastor of 31 years who would lose it all due to his sexual addiction and bad choices – *knowing everything that I would do, God called me to preach anyway.*

I came to Christ at age 14, was called to preach at 15, took my first church position at 19, and became a senior pastor at 24. So when I was 15, God looked at me and, seeing (a) who I was, (b) who I would become, and (c) all that I would do, concluded, "That's the kind of a guy I want to pastor three churches over 31 years of his life."

Strange reasoning, by most standards. I don't have the space to delve into the "All things work together for good" passage (Romans 8:28) or the "God's gifts and his call are irrevocable" verse (Romans 11:29).

But I do have the space to say three things.

1. Nothing we do will make God love us less.
2. Nothing we do will invalidate God's ability to use us.
3. God uses fallen men more than non-fallen men. (There are no non-fallen men.)

So let this sink in. God chose you, Jesus died for you, and the Father longs to bless and use you, not despite the fact that you got off the rails somewhere, but with the full knowledge that you would make bad choices. It's not that your mess doesn't matter. It does. In fact, it matters a lot. But here's the thing—God's providence, purpose, and power are much bigger than that.

Day 5
Am I an Addict?

A lot of guys are okay admitting they have a "struggle." But they resist saying, "I'm an addict." So let's delve into that.

Are you really an addict?

The American Society of Addiction Medicine has identified three descriptors of addiction:

1. Loss of personal control

2. Compulsive activity
3. Continued activity despite harm

Do you view pornography, search for women or men online, or find yourself doing things you don't want to do—repeatedly? Do you continue to do these things despite negative consequences? Then you are probably an addict.

This brings us to Step 1. When you can say it and know it's true, you are on the right road:

"I am powerless over lust—and my life has become unmanageable."

You're in good company. The great apostle wrote, "For I do not the good I want to do, but the evil I do not want to do—this I keep on doing" (Romans 7:15).

Day 6
Blame It on the Native Americans

Comedian Pat Paulsen said, "All of the problems we face today can be traced to the lax immigration policy of the Native Americans."

Paulsen has a point. "All have sinned" (Romans 3:23). That means we all have something going on. Let me demonstrate.

- 14% have a substance addiction. (Surgeon General)
- 77% suffer from stress. (American Institute of Stress)
- 30% suffer from chronic pain. (cdc.gov)
- 7% are clinically depressed. (Healthline)
- 58% have no savings. (Finance.yahoo)
- 38% will get cancer. (National Cancer Institute)
- 33% have high blood pressure. (American Heart Association)
- 50% are overweight. (Healthdate.org)
- 20% have mental illnesses. (NAMI)

Add it up—327 percent of us will have problems with substance abuse, high levels of stress, chronic pain, depression, no savings, cancer, high blood pressure, obesity, and mental illness.

That's a clear majority. Here's the point. If you are struggling with life on some level, you are not alone. In fact, being alone is the problem. It's called isolating. And it feeds, among other things, sex addiction.

Yes, you have problems. We all do. Blame it on the Native Americans. Blame it on your parents. Blame it on whomever you like. But admit that—along with 327 percent of those around you—you have a problem.

Day 7
Acceptance

The hardest step for most addicts is acceptance. Before I got into recovery, I said it a thousand times. "I can do this on my own; I can stop these destructive behaviors when I'm ready."

After all, I have four degrees, planted a church, pastored three churches, was a university board chairman, picked the best wife in the world, and we raised the best son in the world. And while I'm no natural mechanic, I taught myself to change my oil, my radiator, and my valve cover gaskets. I could change everything—except myself.

I just couldn't accept the fact that I am powerless. But that's where God comes in.

The Bible offers great encouragement for those of us who accept our powerlessness. "As a father has compassion on his children, so the Lord has compassion on those who fear him; for he knows how we are formed, he remembers that we are dust" (Psalm 103:13-14).

Psychotherapist Nathaniel Branden said, "The first step toward change is awareness."

That is why we need to echo the prayer attributed to Reinhold Niebuhr every day. "God grant me the serenity to accept the things I cannot change . . ."

You can't address a problem you have not yet accepted. Your only hope is to accept today what you can start working on tomorrow.

Week 2
Boundaries

"Boundaries define us. They define what is me and what is not me. A boundary shows me where I end and someone else begins, leading me to a sense of ownership. Knowing what I am to own and take responsibility for gives me freedom."

- Henry Cloud

THIS WEEK'S EXERCISE
Try Three Boundaries

Your recovery is only as strong as the boundaries you put in place. There are dozens of boundaries that you might need to put in place. And each of us has a different set of boundaries to consider. While we will focus on three boundaries with this exercise, you will need to consult your sponsor, therapist, accountability partner, and/or spouse, as you identify further boundaries that will help keep you safe

Boundary #1—Your Eyes

While we will address the 3-second rule (bounce your eyes) in another segment of this workbook, our interest here is in what you do with your eyes when you are with someone of the opposite sex. Let me speak to guys, specifically. When talking to a woman, look her in the eyes. Do not look at body parts—only her eyes. Even a glance toward a woman's body will get you into trouble, and it devalues her as a human being.

This week, take note of the instances in which you are successful at looking a woman in her eyes, and also note the instances in which you fail. In order to make progress, you need to see how you are really doing in this area.

Women at whom I looked only in the eyes this week:

- _____
- _____
- _____
- _____
- _____
- _____
- _____
- _____
- _____

Women at whom I looked at body parts instead of their eyes:

- _____
- _____
- _____
- _____
- _____
- _____
- _____
- _____
- _____
- _____

Boundary #2—Television

Television presents some real dilemmas for sex addicts. The current pop culture is a highly sexual one. The increase of sexually explicit scenes, jokes, innuendoes, the showing of naked (or near naked) bodies and extramarital activity on television can trigger the addict into a myriad of sexual thoughts and behaviors. Most shows are not a safe place for the person who already struggles with thoughts of sexual fantasy. Below are a series of boundaries you can erect to protect yourself against the dangers of television. Check the boundaries that you will put in place.

- No television for one week _____
- No television for one month _____
- No television without someone else present _____
- Give remote to spouse _____
- No cable television _____
- Watch cable, but only for sports and/or news _____
- No television after 10:00 p.m. _____
- No talk shows _____
- No pay-per-view shows _____
- No Netflix _____
- Other: _____

Boundary #3—The Internet

The Internet is awash with porn sites. The temptations of the Internet are almost limitless. It may be impossible for you to conduct business and live a normal life apart from the Internet. But there are certain boundaries that you can—and must—put in place. Check the boundaries which will work for you, and which you will put in place.

- Get on Covenant Eyes _____
- No Internet at all _____
- No Internet unless someone else is present _____
- No Internet after 10:00 p.m. _____
- No Internet connection to my cell phone _____
- No email use without another person present _____
- No use of Internet in hotel rooms _____
- No Internet at public places _____
- Other: _____

Day 1
Compromise

In politics, business, and marriage, the word for today is compromise. But is compromise all that it's cracked up to be? Sales expert and writer Lisa Earle McLeod wrote, "Refusal to compromise is widely considered to be the root cause of political polarization, business battles, and divorce wars. But refusal to compromise isn't actually the cause of these problems. It's merely a symptom. The real problem is unwillingness to tolerate uncertainty."

Let's talk about compromise. There's a story in the Old Testament you may not recall. The Gibeonites were often at war with Israel. But in an effort to find peace with their more heavily armored foes, the Gibeonites sought to settle in the land adjoining Israel. As a peace offering, they offered samples of their finest goods in order to trick Israel into letting her guard down.

Rather than seeking God in the matter, "The Israelites sampled their provisions but did not inquire of the Lord" (Joshua 9:14). This act of compromise would bring great misery upon God's children.

That's how the enemy works, especially in addiction. Here's his plan: (a) we listen to the offer of compromise, (b) we taste of his provisions, (c) we indulge, and (d) we cohabitate. The next thing you know, we become just like the Gibeonites.

Here's the lesson—don't compromise with the enemy. It never works out.
Stand your ground. Maintain good boundaries. Don't compromise.

Day 2
Hammer and Sword

The Old Testament book of Nehemiah is a template for getting things done. Nehemiah was called by God to rebuild the wall around the holy city of Jerusalem. But it wasn't long before he encountered two men intent on stopping the work: Sanballat and Tobiah, who rallied the forces from Ammon and Ashdod to come against the children of God. The threat to Nehemiah and his work was real.

Nehemiah had to make a decision. Would he stop the work and focus on his enemies? Or would he stay on the job and ignore those who were plotting his destruction?

Nehemiah decided the answer was not either/or, but both/and. He instructed his men to build the wall, while remaining diligent. They literally had a hammer in one hand and a sword in the other.

"Those who carried materials did their work with one hand and held a weapon in the other, and each of the builders wore his sword at his side as he worked" (Nehemiah 4:17-18).

This is exactly how we must walk the road of recovery. We need to move on with the project of rebuilding our lives. But at the same time, we need to keep an eye on the enemy.

You probably have a Sanballat or a Tobiah in your life. They are a threat to good boundaries, and they represent a threat to your sobriety. You must remain diligent in your recovery program, while keeping an eye on the enemy.

Day 3
It Always Starts Small

On September 2, 1666, it started at the home of Thomas Farriner, the king's baker. A fire broke out in Farriner's home, and it quickly spread. Within hours, 80 percent of London had burned to the ground. It is remembered as the Great Fire of London.

Big, tragic events always start small. Consider three events from Scripture.

1. Lot cast his tent "toward Sodom" (Genesis 13:12). It wasn't long before Lot was in Sodom.
2. Peter followed Jesus "from a distance" (Luke 22:54). It wasn't long before Peter denied Christ three times.
3. The youngest son asked his father for his "share of the estate" (Luke 15:12). It wasn't long before he was wasting his life in a far country.

The same is true of addiction. We fall into a hole one tiny step at a time. We don't see it coming. But come it does. I offer three ways to avoid this step-by-step trap.

1. Live one day at a time.
2. Don't assume victory today just because you were good yesterday.
3. Maintain boundaries.

You can stay sober. But you must beware of the traps all around you. One small slip today can result in a mighty fall tomorrow.

Move in the right direction—one small step at a time.

Day 4
The Last Thing Charley Did

A terrible explosion rocked a gunpowder factory. After the mess was cleaned up, the inquiry began. One of the survivors was pulled into the investigator's office and asked, "Okay, Simpson. You were near the scene, so tell me what happened!"

"Well, it was like this, sir. Old Charley Higgins was in the mixing room, and I saw him pull a cigarette from his pocket and light it up."

The investigator responded, "Are you telling me Higgins was smoking in the mixing room? How long had he been with the company?"

"About 20 years, sir."

"Well, he should have known better! You'd think lighting a cigarette in the mixing room would have been the last thing he would do."

"It was, sir."

Here's the lesson. In recovery, our problem is not a lack of knowledge. We are seldom at a loss for what we should avoid in life. Paul wrote, "The acts of the flesh are obvious: sexual immorality, impurity, and debauchery" (Galatians 5:19).

Learn from old Charley Higgins. It's not what you know that matters, but what you do with what you know.

You know the things to do and the things to avoid. Recovery is the alignment of right knowledge and right actions. The next move is yours.

Day 5
Take It from Joe

The story of Joseph is a template for maintaining solid boundaries. Joseph was taken captive to Egypt, where he quickly found favor with the captain of Pharaoh's guard, a man named Potiphar. Potiphar put Joseph in charge of his estate. We read, "Now Joseph was well-built and handsome, and after a while his master's wife took notice of him and said, 'Come to bed with me!'" (Genesis 39:6-8).

That's when things got really crazy. Mrs. Potiphar persisted "day after day" (39:10). Then, when she finally crossed the line and came onto Joseph more aggressively, Joseph ran out of the house (39:12).

Doing the right thing came with a price. First, it meant self-denial, as Joseph denied his fleshly desires in order to do what was right. Second, it cost him a prison term, as Potiphar's wife accused him of a sexual advance.

But cutting off toxic relationships is always the wise thing to do. For Joseph, it meant finding God's favor in prison and emerging stronger than ever. For you, when you cut off relationships with acting out partners or anyone else who feeds your addiction, you will soon find a freedom and peace you never knew.

Day 6
A Second Wall

"Then Hezekiah worked hard at repairing all the broken sections of the wall, erecting towers, and constructing a second wall outside the first" (2 Chronicles 32:5).

In Hezekiah's day, each city was fortified by walls that protected them from outside attack. If these walls became weak or faulty, this left the city in danger of invasion from the enemy. When Hezekiah was king, an enemy was threatening to attack. The king responded by ordering a complete repair of all broken sections, as well as the erection of a second wall.

For us, these walls represent the boundaries we set for ourselves to secure our own protection. Recovery involves two things—repairing weak walls and erecting new ones.

Let's break that down. How are your current walls holding up? Are there any parts of your recovery plan that need to be revisited? Perhaps you are slipping in your attendance at meetings, making recovery calls, or working the steps.

And what about new boundaries? When was the last time you added a layer of recovery work to your routine? This might include listening to certain podcasts or reading recovery literature.

If you wait until the wall comes down, it's too late. I suggest you go the extra mile. Rebuild your current walls. Then build some more.

Repair your first wall of defense. Then start building a second wall.

Day 7
The Enemy Will Find You

During a battle in the Civil War, one of General Longstreet's officers approached him to say that he couldn't obey Longstreet's order to bring up his men to the line of battle, as the enemy was too strong. Longstreet responded with sarcasm. "Very well. Never mind. Just let them stay where they are. The enemy will advance, and that will spare you the trouble."

If we are to maintain sobriety, we must engage the enemies of our recovery every day: temptation, fantasy, past failures, and—most of all—complacency.

An Alpine guide died on a mountainside in Europe. At that spot a sign reads, "He died climbing." May that be said of each of us.

A.W. Tozer said, "Complacency is a deadly foe of all spiritual growth. Acute desire must be present or there will be no manifestation of Christ to his people. He waits to be wanted."

Solomon was right: "Through laziness, the rafters sag; because of idle hands, the house leaks" (Ecclesiastes 10:18).

Engage the enemy or the enemy will engage you. Complacency is not an option. If your house is leaking, it's time to plug the hole.

Your problem is not lack of knowledge, but lack of action. You know what to do. Now do what you know.

Week 3
Structure

"Inside the Bible's pages lie all the answers to all of the problems man has ever known. It is my firm belief that the enduring values presented in its pages have a great meaning for each of us and for our nation. The Bible can touch our hearts, order our minds, and refresh our souls."

- Ronald Reagan

THIS WEEK'S EXERCISE
Developing Your Personal Recovery Plan

The old adage is true—by failing to plan you are planning to fail. Recovery doesn't just happen. Show me a man or woman with long term sobriety and I'll show you a man or woman who is following a plan.

This is true in all aspects of life. Every athlete has a structured workout regimen. Every scholar maintains a lifelong plan of learning. Every successful businessman sets forth a plan for growth and prosperity.

And successful recovery follows a structured plan.

Without a plan, you go through life reacting. Recovery is proactive—always. So write down your personal recovery plan. It will be unlike anyone else's, customized to your specific needs and goals. Write out at least three specific action steps for your personal recovery—daily, weekly, monthly, and yearly.

What I Will Do Every Day

- _____
- _____
- _____
- _____
- _____

What I Will Do Every Week

- _____
- _____
- _____
- _____
- _____

What I Will Do Every Month

- _____
- _____
- _____
- _____
- _____

What I Will Do Every Year

- _____
- _____
- _____
- _____
- _____

Day 1
Pac-Man

I had three majors in college:

1. Christianity
2. Speech
3. Pac-Man

You may have played this most popular video game a thousand times. But did you ever stop to ask yourself, "Where did Toru Iwatani, the creator of Pac-Man, get his inspiration for the shape of the Pac-Man character?"

Pizza.

Iwatani was eating pizza one day, and when he removed the first slice, the image before him stuck in his mind. From that moment, Iwatani dreamed of a video game featuring that image.

It's good to have dreams. It's so good, in fact, that God promised that his children would dream dreams (Amos 2:28).

As you dream of a life of recovery, I suggest you ask yourself two questions.

1. What would my life be like without this addiction?
2. What can I do that I haven't done already?

Recovery is a dream that can come true—if you establish a structure that feeds that dream. Otherwise, the nightmare will continue.

Day 2
Taking It to the Grave

Author Roald Dahl died in 1990 and was buried in a churchyard in Buckinghamshire, England. That part makes sense. But it was what was buried along with Dahl that makes the story interesting. He was buried with his power saw, favorite pencils, and snooker cues.

And chocolate.

Roald Dahl wasn't just any author. He wrote *Charlie and the Chocolate Factory*. The idea of taking one's stuff to the grave isn't new. But it is dumb.

The richest man alive nailed it: "Riches do not last forever" (Proverbs 27:24).

Dr. Edward J. Khantzian wrote a great article, *Insights on the Insanity of Addiction*. He wrote, "A primary factor that contributes to addiction is that the behavior temporarily relieves the emotional pain."

We can become so used to self-medicating with our addictive behaviors that this becomes all we know. Sadly, it may even follow us to the grave.

God has a better plan. If we seek him and we commit to recovery, we will find a peace that diminishes the value of stuff to the point that taking this stuff with us to the grave will never cross our minds.

Day 3
Unchained

Neil Armstrong said, "The important achievement of Apollo was demonstrating that humanity is not forever chained to this planet and our opportunities are unlimited."

Sam Cooke wrote these lyrics to his most famous song:

That's the sound of the men working on the chain gang.
That's the sound of the men working on the chain gang.
All day they work so hard
Till the sun is goin' down.
Working on the highways and byways
And wearing a frown.
You hear them moanin' their lives away,
Then you hear somebody say,
That's the sound of the men working on the chain gang.

Jesus met a man who was part of a chain gang. "This man lived in the tombs, and no one was able to bind him anymore, not even with a chain" (Mark 5:3). Then Jesus set him free.

Are you bound by chains today? Join the gang. But the chain gang has no permanent membership. What Neil Armstrong said of the Apollo space mission rings true for you. You can be freed from your chains, and the opportunities are unlimited.

Day 4
Mulligan

Have you heard of a mulligan? It's a free shot in golf, claimed by millions of hackers across the globe every day. In most friendly competition, each golfer is given one mulligan per 18 holes. But did you know where the term "mulligan" came from?

About 90 years ago, a Canadian golfer named David Bernard Mulligan was playing with three buddies. On the first hole, Mulligan's tee shot missed the fairway badly, sailing into the woods. He did what every self-respecting golfer always does. He made excuses for the horrible shot. His partners gave him a do-over, and the "mulligan" was born.

God is in the mulligan business. None of us would be here without taking more than our fair share of mulligans in life.

In the Old Testament, God's children had strayed off the fairway of life deep into the woods. And they suffered the consequences. But a loving God offered a mulligan.

"I will repay you for the years the locusts have eaten—the great locust and the young locust, the other locusts and the locust swarm—my great army that I sent among you" (Joel 2:25).

Gordon MacDonald wrote, "If our yesterdays are in a state of good repair, they provide strength for today. If not repaired, they create havoc."

You and I need to be repaired. We need a mulligan. We need God.

Day 5
Pushing Trains

Do you ever tire of maintaining the structure of your recovery? Perhaps you can relate to the rural pastor.

The pastor was spotted sitting by the train track each morning. A church member asked him what he was doing. "Why do you sit here watching the train each day?" she asked him.

"It's simple," replied the pastor. "I enjoy watching something move that I don't have to push."

Life is most effective when we leave the pushing to God. The psalmist wrote, "The Lord is my strength and my shield; my heart trusts in him, and he helps me. My heart leaps for joy, and with my song I praise him" (Psalm 28:7).

J.I. Packer said it perfectly: "Our high and privileged calling is to do the will of God in the power of God for the glory of God."

It is natural to want to do all the pushing ourselves. But it doesn't work. We need to learn to let go and let the Conductor take over.

Day 6
Shelter

Jonah was us—each of us. He ran *from God* (chapter 1), *to God* (chapter 2), *with God* (chapter 3), then *ahead of God* (chapter 4). We have all done the same. Toward the end of the story, Jonah isolated. He went off by himself in the depths of depression, where he sat under a tree, which became his shelter of choice. And then we read this:

"At dawn the next day God provided a worm, which chewed the plant so that it withered. When the sun rose, God provided a scorching east wind, and the sun blazed on Jonah's head so that he grew faint. He wanted to die, and said, 'It would be better for me to die than to live'" (Jonah 4:7-8).

The tree became Jonah's crutch. He had come to rely on it for comfort and protection in the midst of his pain. As with Jonah, our addictions function as a shelter from our pain. And as with Jonah, when that crutch is removed, it reveals deep wounds. For Jonah, it was anger. He was angry that God didn't do things the way he wanted, and that his life had not turned out according to his plan.

Sound familiar?

In 1719, Isaac Watts penned these words: *"Our God, our help in ages past, our hope for years to come, our shelter from the stormy blast, and our eternal home."*

Your life has not turned out exactly as you had hoped. No one's does. That leaves you two choices: get bitter or get better. You get better by trusting in the true shelter . . . starting today.

Day 7
Special Delivery

"Then the Lord said to Joshua, 'See, I have delivered Jericho into your hands, along with its king and its fighting men'" (Joshua 6:2).

God is in the delivery business. And the same God who delivered Jericho can deliver you—from your fears, resentments, and addictions. God is the master of accomplishing the unattainable.

Wilbur Howard wrote, "The future belongs to those who set their sights on what is humanly unattainable."

Let me illustrate.

When the World's Fair came to Canada in 1986, Henry Blackaby saw an opportunity to reach more than 22 million people with the message of the gospel. There was just one problem. The association of churches Blackaby served in Vancouver had just 2,000 members and a budget of less than $9,000 a year. Still, convinced of God's leading, Blackaby set a budget of $202,000, prayed and trusted God to do the rest. God didn't disappoint. By the end of the year, more than $264,000 had come in from all over the world, and some 20,000 people began personal relationships with Christ through the efforts of a small but faithful band of believers.

It may feel like you will never be able to quit your porn habit, affairs, or self-stimulation. But the God who delivered the entire city of Jericho stands ready to deliver you—if you let him.

Surrender to the God who is in the delivery business. The next miracle can be yours.

Week 4
Gratitude

"It is only with gratitude that we become rich."

- Dietrich Bonhoeffer

THIS WEEK'S EXERCISE
Thank God for Your Addiction

When attending SA or SAA meetings, I often state that I am grateful for my addiction. The reason is simple. It is my addiction that drove me into a deeper dependence upon God than I had ever known before. My addiction did for me what my church, Christian college, and seminary could not do. It reminded me of my utter helplessness in living a life of power, freedom, and a sound mind.

A sign of true recovery is that you begin to thank God *for* your addiction, rather than *despite* your addiction.

In today's exercise, list the blessings that your struggles have brought into your life. Then write a short letter to God, thanking him for those struggles and for your addiction.

What my addiction has taught me:

1. _____
2. _____
3. _____
4. _____
5. _____

My letter of gratitude to God: _____

_____

_____

_____

_____

_____

_____

_____

_____

Day 1
The Great Philosopher

That great philosopher Willie Nelson said, "When I started counting my blessings, my whole life turned around."

I'll say something I rarely say. Willie makes sense. The fact is, the people who have received the most blessings, who have been healed of the greatest addictions, should be the most grateful for their new lease on life.

Case in point—Mary Magdalene.

Mary was a shining example of gratitude. Once possessed by seven demons, she had been set free by Christ. And she responded with unparalleled gratitude and loyalty. When Jesus was crucified on the cross, she was there. When Jesus needed a tomb for burial, she was there. And when he rose the third day, she was there. She had come to the tomb to offer a sacrifice of rare perfume.

The Bible says, "When Jesus rose early on the first day of the week, he appeared first to Mary Magdalene, out of whom he had driven seven demons" (Mark 16:9). People full of gratitude find themselves at the right place at the right time.

What can you offer God today, in gratitude for the healing he has brought to your life?

Day 2
Satisfaction

There is really only one reason we ever get in trouble. We buy into the false narrative that we need something more in order to be truly satisfied.

A man explained why he bought a new car. "I was faced with the choice of buying a $50 battery for my old car or a new car for $50,000. And they wanted cash for the battery."

Jay Leno was once asked why he had 300 classic cars. He said, "Because 200 wasn't enough." That's the American dream, isn't it? I'm not satisfied with what I have, so I must need more of it.

The Bible offers a different way. "Be satisfied with what you have" (Hebrews 13:5).

G.K. Chesterton said it like this: "There are two ways to get enough. One is to accumulate more. The other is to desire less."

Addiction is a progressive disease. At first, you don't even know you have it. The patient never notices when his temperature hits 98.7. The addict takes in a glance here, a second look there. He watches an "R" movie, becomes casual on the Internet, and pretty soon, he has crossed over to a world he never knew. And what satisfied yesterday no longer does it for him today.

Satisfaction is not a destination, but a choice. If you are tired of crossing all the wrong boundaries, choose satisfaction. If you are tired of grabbing what you were never intended to have, only to find it's never enough, choose satisfaction.

"Be satisfied with what you have" (Hebrews 13:5). It really is enough.

Day 3
Hiding Place

When I was a child, I loved to play "hide and seek." Somehow, no matter how well I thought I had hidden, my father could always find me. Perhaps it was my feet sticking out from under the curtains or my giggling from under the bed covers that gave me away. But in my mind, if I couldn't see my father, he probably couldn't see me.

The good news for every believer is that even when we can't see our Father, he still sees us. King David went through this kind of struggle often—sometimes of his own doing, but not always. He was often overcome with hopelessness and despair.

And then he looked up. And he said this: "The Lord is my rock, my fortress, and my deliverer" (2 Samuel 22:2). And then David found the God who had already found him.

In the past, we used our addiction as our hiding place when life became overwhelming. Now that we are in recovery, life can at times feel even more overwhelming. We need a new place of refuge to escape the storms and find protection.

Philip Yancey wrote, "A God wise enough to create me and the world I live in is wise enough to watch out for me."

Turn to God with a grateful heart, as the one who delights in watching out for you. You've played "hide and seek" long enough. You lost. God won. And that's a good thing.

Day 4
Paid in Full

Søren Kierkegaard wrote, "In the understanding of the moment, never has anyone accomplished so little by the sacrifice of a consecrated life as did Jesus Christ. And yet in this same instant, eternally understood, he had accomplished all, and on that account said, 'It is finished.'"

Peter said that Jesus died to secure "the genuineness of our faith" (1 Peter 1:7).

Jesus' death was not primarily for the history books. It is more personal than that. Because Jesus died for our shortcomings, we can find victory. Freedom is not based on what we can do, but on what he has already done.

In the nineteenth century, Elvina Hall understood this when she became the first person to perform a new hymn, at the Monument Street Methodist Church in Baltimore. This is the first stanza of that hymn. Perhaps you've heard of it.

I heard the Savior say, thy strength indeed is small.
Child of weakness, watch and pray, find in me thine all in all.
Jesus paid it all, all to him I owe;
Sin had left a crimson stain, he washed it white as snow.

Jesus paid it all, then said, "It is finished." That means we can live *from* victory, not *for* victory. And we can do so with grateful hearts.

Day 5
How Sober People Are Different

What is the difference between people who are sober and those who aren't?

Kelly Fitzgerald addresses this question in her article, The 7 Biggest Differences Between Sober People and Normies. She writes, "Our gratitude levels are different. Through recovery I have learned to be grateful for each moment and for waking up each day sober and alive. When you've been to hell and back, your gratitude levels run pretty deep."

The Psalmist declared, "Those who look to him for help will be radiant with joy; no shadow of shame will darken their faces" (Psalm 34:5).

Shame for joy—not a bad trade! The key is gratitude, which turns our focus away from ourselves. This theme is captured in the words of George Orwell: "Men can only be happy when they do not assume that the object of life is happiness."

If you continue to struggle with sobriety, try this. Practice gratitude—then wait. Joy is on the way.

If you are ready to trade shame for joy, I offer a very simple idea. Make a gratitude list. Then pray off of this list, expressing thanks to God for all of his blessings.

Day 6
Joanna

You remember Joanna of the Bible, don't you? If not, let me refresh your memory.

This ignored Bible character was actually quite a woman. We read her story in Luke 8 and Luke 23–24. Joanna was healed of evil spirits by Jesus. She later supported him and his disciples in their travels. Joanna, whose name means "God is gracious," stayed with Jesus through the crucifixion and later became one of the three women who visited his tomb early on Easter morning.

Joanna's last appearance in the Bible is recorded: "It was Mary Magdalene, Joanna, Mary the mother of James, and the others with them who told this (news of the resurrection) to the apostles" (Luke 24:10).

Joanna is a significant person in the Bible because she simply brought good news to others. By her personal testimony, she encouraged others to walk straighter paths and lead fuller lives, which would not have been possible apart from the power of the resurrection.

Step 12 is about helping others. Your recovery is not complete until you take the message of sobriety to others. God wants to do *through you* what he has already done *to you*.

Day 7
Hold the Rope

In 1792, William Carey committed to a dangerous life of mission work in India. When many questioned his sanity, he recruited his closest friends to support him and his efforts. He said, "I will descend into the pit, but only if you hold tightly to the ropes."

Sometimes, the only thing more painful than falling into the pit of addiction is crawling out. One of the most common mistakes an addict—new to recovery—can make is to try to do it alone. But if no one above is holding the other end of the rope, the rope is of no use. And the addict will remain trapped.

The Bible speaks of God's blessing on those who help the fallen. "God will not forget your work and the love you have shown him as you have helped his people and continue to help them" (Hebrews 6:10).

Let me suggest four things you can do to help your friend rise from the pit of addiction.

1. Give her your time.
2. Give her your shoulder.
3. Give her your experience.
4. Give her your prayers.

If you don't know someone who is new to recovery, you need to go to more meetings. Here's my challenge. At your next 12-Step meeting, focus not on your buddies whom you know well, but on the man or woman who is new to recovery. They are in the pit. And you hold the rope.

Week 5
Spiritual Connection

*"To fall in love with God is the greatest romance; to seek
him the greatest adventure; to find him,
the greatest human achievement."*

\- Saint Augustine

THIS WEEK'S EXERCISE
Write a Letter to God

Successful recovery is spiritual recovery. Any 12-Step group speaks often of a "higher power," even if they whiff on defining who this "higher power" is. You cannot maintain long-term sobriety apart from your connection to God.

In a moment, you will write a letter to God. But first, let's dig a little deeper. How did your spiritual connection evolve to where it is today?

In what ways did your mother model a spiritual connection?

_____

_____

_____

_____

_____

How did your father demonstrate a spiritual connection?

_____

_____

_____

_____

_____

How have your parents' spiritual beliefs and practices affected you personally?

_____

_____

How can you avoid the negative influences of your parents' spiritual shortfalls?

_____

_____

_____

_____

_____

Describe your relationship with God as a child:

_____

_____

_____

_____

_____

How has your relationship with God evolved since childhood?

_____

_____

_____

_____

How have your addiction and recovery affected your spiritual connection?

_____

_____

_____

_____

_____

Write a letter to God. Tell him how you would like your spiritual connection to evolve in the coming days.

_____

_____

_____

_____

_____

_____

_____

_____

Day 1
God's Clean vs. Our Dirty

God's clean overcomes our dirty.

Jesus' first miracle occurred at a wedding. They had run out of wine and didn't know what to do. So they turned to Jesus. We all know the end of the story. Jesus turned the water into wine and saved the day.

But don't miss how he did it. Notice his instrument of choice.

"Nearby stood six stone water jars, used for Jewish ceremonial washing. Each could hold twenty to thirty gallons" (John 2:6).

These were not clean jars. And Jesus didn't clean them up before he used them. But the wine came out fine. How did this happen?

God's clean overcomes our dirty.

In recovery—and in life—we often get this idea that we must become clean so God can use us. Actually, it works the other way. When God uses us, we become clean. Yes, we need to practice the spiritual disciplines that lead to a life of righteousness—Bible reading, prayer, etc. But if we wait until we are completely clean to be used, we will never be used. Say it with me . . .

God's clean overcomes our dirty.

Day 2
Give It a Rest

God did not create us to be human *doings*. We are human *beings*. Still, most of us are driven to success, as measured by others. This requires crazy hours, leaving little time for much else. Things that really matter are crowded out of our lives. Too often, recovery work is the first to go.

Enter this famous verse: "Be still, and know that I am God" (Psalm 46:10).

For most of us, being still does not come easily. Fortunately, many therapists and doctors are now recognizing the benefits of rest.

I came across one article titled, *86 Benefits of Stillness with God.*

Alex Soojung-Kim Pang wrote in his helpful book, *Rest*, that rest has been proven to make us more effective at work.

And celebrity nutritionist Kimberly Snyder adds, "Our society puts too much emphasis on constant doing, without recognizing that in the recharging space you can come back to work, duties and relationships in a more productive, enhanced way."

The evidence is in. Rest is a good thing. It allows us to recharge, reflect, and renew. If you are too busy for rest, then you are just too busy.

Make time for this verse today. "Be still, and know that I am God."

Day 3
Your Most Compelling Goal

J.I. Packer wrote, "What makes life worthwhile is having a big enough objective, something which catches our imagination and lays hold of our allegiance; and this the Christian has in a way that no other person has. For what higher, more exalted, and more compelling goal can there be than to know God?"

Jim Elliot said it like this: "Oh, the fullness, pleasure, sheer excitement of knowing God on earth!"

All successful recovery connects the addict to his Higher Power. The prophet wisely declared, "I desired the knowledge of God more than burnt offerings" (Hosea 6:6).

I like to say it like this—*seek recovery and you will be frustrated; seek God and recovery will find you.*

The problem for so many of us is that while we want recovery and long to know God, we cling to our old habits, as well. Why is this? To quote C.S. Lewis, "The problem is, we are too easily pleased."

It's time to raise the bar. It's time to no longer be so "easily pleased." It's time to find real recovery. It's time to find God.

Day 4
Big Boys Do Cry

U.S. military chaplain William Thomas Cummings preached a sermon during the Battle of Bataan in 1942, in which he allegedly said, "There are no atheists in a foxhole." While there has been no official corroboration that he actually spoke those words, this seems to be the origin of that common phrase.

Hear God's invitation: "Call on me in the day of trouble; I will deliver you, and you will honor me" (Psalm 50:15). The word used for "call" means to cry to God with a desperate voice.

Nothing has a man in deeper trouble than sex addiction. But what is the significance of crying out to God in such times of trouble? I see three things.

1. This cry represents humility. When you cry to God, you are not bargaining; you are admitting your absolute powerlessness over your addiction.
2. This is a time of surrender. By crying out to God, you are releasing your will to his. You are confessing your total reliance upon God.
3. This is a cry for mercy. By throwing yourself onto the care of God, you are asking for his deliverance, which cannot be earned or deserved.

Your addiction has you in a hole. It's time to crawl out of that hole. But you can't do it on your own. It's time to cry out to God.

Day 5
Spiritual Awakening

We read an interesting passage in the Old Testament. "The hand of the Lord was on me, and he brought me out by the Spirit of the Lord and set me in the middle of a valley; it was full of bones . . . bones that were very dry . . . The Lord said, 'I will put my Spirit in you and you will live, and I will settle you in your land. Then you will know that I the Lord have spoken, and I have done it, declares the Lord'" (Ezekiel 37:1-2, 17).

God brought his prophet Ezekiel to the valley of dry bones. Then God promised these bones would come to life again. The story is one of a spiritual awakening—an awakening that would give hope to God's children.

Philosopher Teilhard de Chardin was right: "We are not human beings having a spiritual experience. We are spiritual beings having a human experience."

The sooner we recognize our spiritual existence, the sooner we will find successful recovery.

Step 11 says it like this: "We sought through prayer and meditation to improve our conscious contact with God, as we understood him, praying only for knowledge of his will for us and the power to carry that out."

You cannot overcome your personal struggles apart from a spiritual connection. Take time today to connect with God through prayer and meditation.

Day 6
Five Powerful Words

There was a young man in the Bible named Hezekiah. He was raised in a dysfunctional home. His father was King Ahaz of Judah, who set up idols for the people to worship. Because he didn't honor God, the nation went downhill and became very poor. Five different armies came against Judah, and Judah lost every battle. The place was decimated. You would think that Ahaz would have learned his lesson, turned to God, and asked for his help, but he did the opposite. He closed the doors of the temple and began to sell off sacred treasures.

Hezekiah was raised in this environment of compromise, defeat, and mediocrity. He could have turned out like his dad; he could have adapted to that environment. But when he became king, the first thing Hezekiah did, before repairing the roads or getting the economy going, was to reopen the temple. He turned the nation back toward God.

His father chose to compromise and to push people down, but Hezekiah's attitude was, "I might have been born in the land of mediocrity, but I'm not going to live there."

What made Hezekiah great? Despite the example of his father, "Hezekiah trusted in the Lord" (2 Kings 18:5).

Those five words are a mouthful. "Hezekiah trusted in the Lord."

Like King Hezekiah, you may have been raised by a father who did not seek the Lord. Did that make life harder for you? Definitely. Did it feed your addiction? Probably. But did it seal a destiny of compromise and failure? Absolutely not.

Day 7
Home

Dignitaries lined the street when the funeral procession passed. Thousands waited just to catch a glimpse of the coffin. In fact, the people of the United States and all parts of the world loved and revered the deceased man so much that his remains were disinterred in Tripoli and brought to the United States for a magnificent funeral.

His name was John Howard Payne. You probably haven't heard of him. But you have probably heard of one line which he famously penned.

"Mid pleasures and palaces, though oft I may roam,

Be it ever so humble; there's no place like home."

Addicts are seeking a home—a place of tranquility. Their addiction has become a familiar friend. But deep down, they know this is not home; it's just a cheap place to rent, and the rent keeps going up. Worse, it is never quite as comfortable as advertised.

God has a better plan. He declared, "I know the plans I have for you, plans to prosper you and not to harm you, plans to give you hope and a future" (Jeremiah 29:11).

You are seeking something or somebody. We all are. But what you really want is a home—a place of safety and peace. And you can find that, but only in Christ.

Week 6
Discipline

"Discipline is the bridge between goals and accomplishments."

- Jim Rohn

THIS WEEK'S EXERCISE
Identifying Your Weakest Link

Your recovery is no stronger than your weakest link.

Everyone has a weakness. We all have at least one habit, character flaw, or personal challenge we must overcome in order to maintain sobriety. This may be tied to the roots of our addiction—abuse, trauma, or isolation. In some cases, it is impossible to trace the genesis of this "weak link." But it is there, and it keeps tripping us up—over and over.

I have known dozens of men who followed solid recovery plans, but still fell to chronic slips and relapses. Why? Because they never dealt with their weakest link.

I've seen other men frustrated by their inability to stay on track with their recovery. The culprit? Their weakest link.

Your weakest link may be known only to you. It may fall into one of the following categories, or none at all:

- Triggers
- Certain types of people
- Past memories
- Euphoric recall
- Fantasy
- Certain places
- Making calls
- Attending meetings
- A specific temptation

Your task this week is to do two things: (a) identify the weakest link in your recovery, and (b) do something about it.

What is the weakest link to your personal recovery?

_____

_____

_____

_____

What will you do to address it this week?

_____

_____

_____

_____

_____

Day 1
Deciding Is Not Enough

Five frogs sat on a log. Three decided to jump off. How many remained on the log? Answer: five. Here's the thing. *Deciding* to do something and *actually doing* it aren't the same thing.

A million times, I decided to stop acting out in my addiction. But I didn't really stop. Why? Because decision and action are two different things.

James warned his readers, "Be doers of the Word, and not hearers only, deceiving yourselves" (James 1:22).

Addiction is all about deception. We deceive ourselves into thinking we can stop anytime, that we are really in control, that we don't need God's help. And when we decide to stop our destructive routines, we think that this decision will be enough.

Decisions are not enough. They must be followed by action.

Zig Ziglar said, "It was character that got us out of bed, commitment that moved us into action, and discipline that enabled us to follow through."

Every addict needs that discipline. Decide to be sober and in recovery. Then do something about it. Follow through: go to meetings, pray, get a sponsor, seek God daily.

Are you ready for real recovery? Then get off the log. It's time to jump!

Day 2
Self-Control

A man was standing in line at a grocery store check-out when he witnessed a man struggling to control his son, about two years of age. The boy was trying to grab everything in sight and toss it into the shopping cart. The dad kept repeating, "Just be calm, Albert. Don't act up, Albert. Don't make a scene, Albert. Control yourself, Albert. Don't act like a child, Albert."

The bystander approached the man with praise. "Sir, I couldn't help but overhear you. I just want to say how impressed I am with the way you just handled little Albert."

The man responded, "Sir, the boy's name is Jimmy. My name is Albert."

Albert is like most of us. We have a much easier time controlling others than ourselves. We are like Lucy, who told Charlie Brown, "I plan to change the world—starting with you."

In recovery, whereas there are principles to be embraced, Scriptures to be read, meetings to be attended, and steps to be followed, there is this one thing we all must have.

Self-control.

The good news is self-control is prayed down, not worked up. It is the result of a spiritual connection. Paul wrote, "The Holy Spirit produces this kind of fruit in our lives: love, joy, peace, patience, kindness, goodness, faithfulness, gentleness, and *self-control*" (Galatians 5:22-23).

You can't make it without good old-fashioned self-control. And you find that in God.

Day 3
The Silver Bullet

Is there a silver bullet to sobriety? Is there one key, one thing that will bring recovery? Is there a simple fix?

The answer is yes, but you aren't going to like what it is. It's called *discipline*.

Paul told young Timothy how to win in life. "Fight the good fight of the faith" (1 Timothy 6:12).

I've seen boxers fight and I've seen them train. The fight is determined by the training. It is the miles of roadwork and hundreds of rounds in the gym that create the successful fighter. It is what is done when no one is watching that makes the fighter great.

In your addiction, you have found your strongest opponent. He will come at you with everything that he's got. And he keeps getting up, no matter how many rounds you have won. He is relentless in his attack and unyielding in his efforts. And even though you may be ahead on points, he can still take you out with a single punch in the final round.

Unless you are diligent in your preparation and disciplined in your defense. Jim Rohn was right: "Discipline is the bridge between goals and accomplishment."

If you are committed to your sobriety, you must embrace the discipline that precedes each battle—discipline to go to meetings, make calls, and never give up.

Day 4
Out of the Zone

Ray Lewis said, "Before anything great is really achieved, your comfort zone must be disturbed."

Ashton Kutcher added, "I'm continually trying to make choices that put me against my own comfort zone. As long as you're uncomfortable, it means you're growing."

We often hear the phrase, "in the zone." We want to live "in the zone," whatever that means. When it comes to the comfort zone, that is the last place an addict needs to live.

Why does an addict return to his old, destructive ways? Because his addiction is his most reliable friend. It is there when he wants it—always available and consistently willing.

The dilemma that faces all who begin to seek sobriety is that they want to feel comfortable. Therefore, they only embrace those recovery activities that are easy, and not challenging. But real recovery takes real courage—to step out, risk being known, and unearth the darkest secrets of one's past.

On the precipice of his greatest challenge, Joshua heard from God: "Have I not commanded you? Be strong and courageous. Do not be frightened, and do not be dismayed, for the Lord your God is with you wherever you go" (Joshua 1:9).

Today, you need to hear from God. The good news is that he has already spoken.

Day 5
The Four Phases of Recovery

Successful recovery is a four-phase process.

Dr. Milton Magness identifies these phases of recovery: survival, stability, sustaining, and freedom. He says the freedom phase rarely kicks in before 2.5 years of recovery. He describes this phase as meeting three criteria: (a) at least one year of unbroken sobriety; (b) living a balanced, growing life; and (c) having reached the point at which acting out has become more of a memory than a temptation.

Recovery, like life, is a process.

When we think of Samuel, of the Old Testament, we often think of the historic figure who would be Israel's last judge and her first prophet. We remember him as the man who anointed both Saul and David, Israel's first two kings. He was a priest and a Nazarite, the author of the 99th Psalm, and one of only eight people in the Bible to whom God spoke by name.

But Samuel wasn't born great. 1 Samuel 2:26 says, "And the boy Samuel continued to grow in stature and in favor with the Lord."

Growing into one's destiny is a process. It cannot be rushed. In recovery, all four phases of recovery—survival, stability, sustaining, and freedom—are to be celebrated.

Day 6
Follow Through

Successful recovery is a full-time enterprise. We must go all in.

A construction crew was putting a drain line in a building. A power cable was directly in the path of their work. Construction stopped while an electrician was called, who declared that there was no electrical power to the cable.

The foreman asked the electrician, "Are you sure the power is dead to the cable and there is no danger?"

The electrician said, "Absolutely. It's safe to cut the line."

The foreman said, "Then *you* cut the line!"

The electrician countered, "Well, I'm not *that* sure!"

Consider Isaiah 43:18-19. "Forget the former things; do not dwell on the past. See, I am doing a new thing!"

Recovery is not about right decisions, but right actions. It's about going all in.

What actions do you need to take in your recovery? Quit making decisions about it. It's time for follow-through. It's time to go all in.

Day 7
Line in the Sand

The date was March 5, 1836. Col. William Travis, age 26, was in charge of 189 other Texans who sought valiantly to defend the Alamo. They were surrounded by 1,500 Mexicans, under the command of General Santa Anna. History tells us that Travis drew a line in the sand with his sword, then addressed his men. "I now want every man who is determined to stay here and die with me to come across this line." All but one joined him on the other side. The next day, they all fell to the enemy. But by delaying Santa Anna's advance to the east, they allowed Sam Houston the time needed to gather enough forces to win the war, and Texas' battle for independence, one month later.

In your battle for sobriety, you need to try it all—therapy, 12-Step work, Covenant Eyes, accountability, prayer, bouncing your eyes, thought replacement, SA, SAA, SLA, and the NBA. But it really boils down to one thing—a line in the sand.

You must decide, "I'll do whatever it takes for as long as it takes." It's what the Bible calls "counting the cost" (Luke 14:28).

It's what I call discipline.

The next time you are tempted to view porn, draw a line in the sand. When you consider masturbating, remember the line in the sand. And when you feel entitled to self-indulgence, return to that line.

Week 7
Fantasy

"What you think, you become."

- Buddha

THIS WEEK'S EXERCISE
Learn from Your Fantasies

This week's exercise will get very personal. This might be a good time to make sure you are keeping this workbook in a safe place! This week's work—and readings—will require you to look deep into your mind and soul, and to bring into the light aspects of your personal thought life that you grasp with a tight fist. This exercise will require you to reveal things that even a CSAT (Certified Sex Addiction Therapist) will not ask you, nor will they be included in a clinical disclosure or polygraph.

Dr. Jay Stringer is right. He has stepped into the arena of fantasy and found that our fantasies say so much about us. In that regard, your deepest, most intimate sexual fantasies are not inherently wrong. They simply paint a picture. And it is that picture that matters.

Let's get to work. This week, revisit this exercise every day. Write down your sexual fantasies, and more importantly, what you think they say about you. This space will not allow for a detailed description of each fantasy, so just record a brief account of each one you can remember at the end of each day.

Fantasy: _____

_____

_____

What it says about me: _____

_____

_____

Fantasy: _____

_____

_____

What it says about me: _____

_____

_____

Fantasy: _____

_____

_____

What it says about me: _____

_____

_____

Fantasy: _____

_____

_____

What it says about me: _____

_____

_____

Fantasy: _____

_____

_____

What it says about me: _____

_____

_____

Fantasy: _____

_____

_____

What it says about me: _____

_____

_____

Day 1
Fantasy

What we think today is what we do tomorrow. And what we do tomorrow is what we become the next day. It all starts in the head. One of the biggest mistakes people make early in their recovery is to minimize their thought lives.

A leading instrument of relapse is sexual fantasy. An interesting study found that for those in therapy, they spend 42 times more time on their phone apps and social media than in their actual therapy. This, of course, opens the mind to all kinds of intrusive thoughts.

What's so bad about fantasy? We find one answer from Israeli psychologist Dr. Gurit E. Birnbaum. In an article posted in the *Personality and Social Psychology Bulletin*, Birnbaum shares her work. She conducted a case study of 48 married couples. She discovered the reason we fantasize. "Sexual fantasy is a way to avoid intimacy."

Paul spoke to this danger with clarity. "Clothe yourself with the presence of the Lord Jesus Christ. And don't let yourself think about ways to indulge evil desires" (Romans 13:14).

You have two choices: fantasy or intimacy. And God's Word is so clear. The better route for each of us is that we not even *think about ways to indulge evil desires.* You can have fantasy or you can have intimacy. But you can't have both. Choose wisely.

Day 2
Build It Up or Tear It Down

Pastor and humorist Charles Lowry is a trained psychologist. Speaking on the subject of sex addiction, he writes, "We either build up the fantasy and tear down reality or we build up reality and tear down the fantasy."

The real definition of sexual sobriety is progressive victory over lust. And lust begins in the mind.

The Bible has a lot to say about the mind. It warns us against impure thoughts. "Finally, brothers, whatever is true, whatever is honorable, whatever is just, whatever is pure, whatever is lovely, whatever is commendable, if there is any excellence, if there is anything worthy of praise, think about these things" (Philippians 4:8).

Fantasy is a huge problem. But there is an answer. The way to rid our minds of impure thoughts is to fill them with pure thoughts. That's how we tear down the fantasy and build up reality.

Buddha was right: "We are shaped by our thoughts; we become what we think." I'm guessing you want to win the battle for purity. It begins in the mind. It begins with your next thought—and then the one after that.

A pure life follows a pure mind. Starting today, fill your mind with those thoughts that are holy and pure.

Day 3
Kryptonite

When I was a kid, I liked to dress up like Superman. I jumped off furniture as if I could fly. I dreamed of powers I didn't really have. Superman was every boy's hero. But even Superman could be brought down—by something called kryptonite. Kryptonite is a fictitious substance from a radioactive element from Superman's home planet of Krypton. When we watched the TV show on Saturday mornings, we couldn't really see the kryptonite, but we knew it was there.

That's how it is with recovery. It's what no one can see that matters. We can do all the right things, attend meetings, say prayers, and have a sponsor. By all outward appearances, we are sober and well.

But we have a kryptonite that nobody else can see. It's called our heart. We are holding onto something—a fantasy, a person, an intrigue. It's deep inside of us. But if left untreated, it is the disease that will bring us down.

Jesus said, "What goes into someone's mouth does not defile them, but what comes out of their mouth, that is what defiles them" (Matthew 15:11).

It's what is going on inside of us that matters most. Ralph Waldo Emerson is credited with these memorable words: "Sow a thought and you reap an action; sow an action and you reap a habit; sow a habit and you reap a character; sow a character and you reap a destiny."

You can learn to fly like Superman—victorious over temptation. But beware of your thought life. That's the kryptonite that can bring you down.

Day 4
Porn on the Brain

Porn sites receive more traffic than Netflix, Amazon, and Twitter combined (HuffPost). Thirty-five percent of all Internet downloads are porn-related (Web-Root). People who admit to extramarital affairs are over 300 percent more likely to be users of pornography (Social Science Quarterly).

That sex and porn addiction are a rapidly growing crisis is not up for debate. God recognized the damage that results from sexual immorality long before the development of the Internet. Two thousand years ago, he warned, "Put to death whatever belongs to your earthly nature: sexual immorality, impurity, lust, evil desires and greed, which is idolatry" (Colossians 3:5).

So if we know this addiction destroys lives, and if we recognize God's standards of purity, why is this such a struggle?

Science offers an answer. Neurosurgeon Donald Hilton explains the effect of porn on the brain: "Pornography causes release of adrenaline from an area in the brain called the locus coeruleus, and this makes the heart race in those who view, or even anticipate, viewing pornography. The sexual pleasure of pornography may be partially caused by release of dopamine from the ventral tegmental area, and this stimulates the nucleus accumbens, one of the key pleasure centers of the brain."

Translation: Your fight for purity and sobriety is not just a battle with your eyes. The struggle is in your head. And though you are in the battle of your life, it is a battle you can win.

Porn is everywhere, including your brain. Your response? Take your temptations seriously, and surrender completely to God.

Day 5
Ritualization Phase

Patrick Carnes gave us the "addiction cycle" in his early writings. This cycle includes the ritualization phase, which Carnes says "hijacks the brain." This is the phase of addiction in which routines are established in order to set the scene and prepare for the next event of acting out.

For many, the ritualization—or planning—phase is as exciting as the culmination of the process. Some spend hours planning their next rendezvous, date, or neighborhood cruise. They save the money, orchestrate the event, and plan every detail.

The Bible warns us, "Put on the Lord Jesus Christ, and don't make plans to gratify the desires of the flesh" (Romans 13:14).

How exactly do we "make plans to gratify the desires of the flesh"? We download the app, subscribe to the magazine, cruise the neighborhood, browse social media, and visit the bar.

I learned years ago that I rarely do what I don't first plan. Acting out doesn't "just happen." To find sobriety, the key is to cut the process off early—in the ritualization phase. Until you think it, you won't do it. The key is to not think it in the first place.

Day 6
A Better Thought Life

If God can raise a dead Jesus, he can help you with your thought life.

And that is where most of us get into trouble—with our thought lives. This is my version of the addiction cycle: (a) think it, (b) plan it, (c) do it, (d) hate it, (e) cover it, (f) do it again. Notice where it always begins—with our thought lives.

Buddha said, "We are shaped by our thoughts; we become what we think. When the mind is pure, joy follows like a shadow that never leaves."

The Bible says it even better: "We demolish arguments and every pretention that sets itself up against the knowledge of God, and we take captive every thought to make it obedient to Christ" (2 Corinthians 10:5).

For very practical advice on how to conquer our thought lives before they conquer us, we turn to Virginia Gilbert, licensed Marriage and Family Therapist. She suggests, "Replace your fantasies and obsessions with meaningful activities. Your fantasy addiction robs you of productivity. So stop wasting time thinking about someone you can't have. Use that time to pursue constructive interests and hobbies: sports, cooking, music, writing, photography, volunteering. Developing skills and interests is a productive use of your time and adds to your personal growth."

Can you overcome your fantasy thought life? Yes! Let's end today where we began. If God can raise a dead Jesus, he can help you with your thought life.

Day 7
A Strange Instructor

Dr. Jay Stringer has released his first book, *Unwanted: How Sexual Brokenness Reveals Our Way to Healing.* The book is a compilation of research conducted on 3,800 men and women. Stringer summarizes, "The research showed that unwanted sexual behavior is not random. It is both shaped and predicted by the parts of our story that remain unaddressed." Then Stringer concludes, "Don't condemn your fantasy; listen to it."

I have neither the space nor the training to fully unpack that statement: "Don't condemn your fantasy; listen to it."

But here is the simple application. One of the surest ways to look deep within to see why you do what you do is to take a second look at your fantasy life.

James warned, "Each person is tempted when he is lured and enticed by his own desire" (1:14). Notice James spoke of each man's *own* desire. My fantasies are different from yours. There is a reason for that—we have different backgrounds, trauma levels, and exposure to shame.

You are a product of your past and the fantasy you struggle with today may be the best window through which you can view that complicated past. Before you write off your fantasies as sinful indulgences of the mind, learn from them. Let your fantasies shine light on the darkest crevices of your past that you might otherwise completely miss.

Week 8
Self-Care

"Love yourself first, and everything else falls in line.
You really have to love yourself to get anything
done in this world.

- Lucille Ball

THIS WEEK'S EXERCISE
Do a Recovery Day

It may have been the best advice my sponsor ever gave me. "Do a Recovery Day."

"What is a Recovery Day?" I asked.

He explained. A Recovery Day is one full day set aside to focus on recovery, spirituality, and self-care. The day is spent alone with God, other than making a few recovery calls and/or attending a recovery meeting. The day features recovery exercises and literature, but also time spent in a healthy place, doing relaxing activities that feed sanity and recovery.

To give you an example of what a Recovery Day might look like, I'll list the things I often include in my own Recovery Day experiences.

- Walk on the beach
- Visit an antique car museum
- Eat at my favorite ice cream shop
- Read recovery material
- Pray
- Attend a recovery meeting
- Drive along the beach
- Find a new lunch place

Your Recovery Day will look different from mine. But the basic components must be in place: solitude, meditation, recovery work, and self-care.

Try to do a Recovery Day this week. If that is impossible, schedule it for a day soon, then finish the exercise at that time.

Date of my Recovery Day: _____

Place for my Recovery Day: _____

Activities for my Recovery Day:

1. _____

2. _____

3. _____

4. _____

5. _____

6. _____

7. _____

Day 1
Desiderata

I love the line in the film *Desiderata* that says, "Behind a wholesome discipline, be gentle to yourself."

When the prophet Elijah was down physically, emotionally, and spiritually, God sent an angel to give him an interesting message. "Get up and eat, for the journey is too much for you" (1 Kings 19:8).

If you are in recovery, you are on a journey that does not end. The message of the angel to Elijah could be the message to every addict: "The journey is too much for you." So what do we do about that? The example of Elijah is simple. Practice self-care. The angel told him to get up and eat.

How can you practice self-care? I offer the following suggestions.

1. Get enough sleep.
2. Eat when you are hungry.
3. Get outside.
4. Talk about your feelings.
5. Accept who you are.
6. Get a hobby.
7. Hang out with friends.
8. Get a dog. (I recommend a Westie!)
9. Pray.

Let's end where we began: "Be gentle to yourself."

Day 2
The Great Jerry Seinfeld

The great theologian Jerry Seinfeld made this observation about life: "Sometimes the road less traveled is less traveled for a reason."

Unfortunately, the road to recovery is a road less traveled. The evidence is in, and it's not good news. According to a study by the Substance Abuse and Mental Health Services Administration in 2018, of the 20.7 million people over the age of 12 who suffer from destructive addictions, only 4 million ever seek help. That means 81% never do.

Translation: 16.7 million addicts have remained on the road most traveled. Why is this? I offer three observations. People don't seek help because . . .

1. The pleasure is greater than the pain.
2. The problem is easier than the solution.
3. The lust is stronger than the loss.

You can give the addict advice, programs, resources, counseling, and the greatest treatment ever produced, but until she is desperate and broken, she will rarely seek help.

You may know someone like this. You have been praying for them. But perhaps you have been praying the wrong prayer. Rather than praying their road becomes easier, maybe you need to pray for things to get rough—so rough that they are willing to take a detour.

To the road less traveled.

Jesus said, "Wide is the road that leads to destruction" (Matthew 7:14). It's time to get on a different road, the road to recovery—the road less traveled.

Day 3
God's Strength

The year was 1911. The South Pole was not the vacation paradise it is today. But a Norwegian explorer named Roald Amundsen changed all that when he set out to become the first man to reach the South Pole. While assembling his team, Amundsen chose expert skiers and dog handlers. His strategy was simple. The dogs would do most of the work as they pulled the group 15 to 20 miles a day. Rather than rely on their own strength, they would rely on the strength of the dogs. It worked, as Amundsen became the first man to reach the South Pole.

The road to recovery is one of exploration. None of us got it right the first time. And as long as we sought sobriety in our own strength, we found no recovery at all.

The key to lasting recovery is surrender to our Higher Power. As Roald Amundsen relied on the strength of his dogs, we must rely on the strength of our God.

King David wrote, "The Lord is the strength of my life; of whom shall I be afraid?" (Psalm 27:1).

The troubles of this life multiply and can become overwhelming—downright scary. And if we don't learn to rely on God's strength, we become gripped by fear.

Alexander MacLaren nailed it when he said, "Only he who can say, 'The Lord is the strength of my life' can also say, 'Of whom shall I be afraid?'"

Day 4
Generational Curse

Israel suffered from a generational curse. "For a long time Israel was without the true God, without a priest to teach and without the law" (2 Chronicles 15:3).

Here's the story.

When Asa assumed the throne as king of Judah, he also inherited a terrible family tradition. For three generations his family had led the nation in the practice of pagan worship, with its accompanying sexual immorality and moral and spiritual decay. Asa knew that changing these long-established practices would alienate him from his relatives. But he determined that pleasing God was more important than pleasing his family. So King Asa destroyed all evidence of idol worship in Israel and repaired the altar of the Lord. He even removed his grandmother from her powerful and influential position as queen. Imagine the flak Asa must have received after making that decision!

Most importantly, Asa led Judah back to worshiping the one true God. He changed the course of his own personal life and in the process the course of an entire nation, for as long as he remained in office.

Perhaps addiction runs in your family. Studies show that sex addict parents tend to have sex addict children. But it doesn't have to be that way.

Robert Strand wrote *Breaking the Generational Curse*. He said, "The sacrifice of Jesus Christ on the cross is strong enough to break any curse." By the power of God, you can break free. Generational curses are real, but so is God's amazing, healing grace.

Day 5
Trauma

Patrick Carnes' study in 1992 found that 97% of addicts were at some point in their past emotionally abused, 87 percent were at some point physically abused, and 82 percent were sexually abused.

Dr. Gabor Mate has written extensively on the role of trauma in sex addiction, with a focus on how trauma relates to the brain and nervous systems and as a catalyst for addiction. He writes, "Not all addictions are rooted in abuse or trauma, but I do believe they can all be traced to painful experience. A hurt is at the center of all addictive behaviors."

I agree that trauma plays a huge role in the development of addiction, both from my research and my personal experience. The question is not whether trauma is at the root of addiction, but how the addict should respond.

Authors at HelpGuide.org have offered several suggestions. Foremost is the insistence that we not isolate.

At this point the psalmist gives us hope. "He will cover you with his pinions, and under his wings you will find refuge; his faithfulness is a shield and buckler. You will not fear the terror of the night, nor the arrow that flies by day, nor the pestilence that stalks in darkness, nor the destruction that wastes at noonday" (Psalm 81:4-6).

If you are an addict, you have trauma in your background—that is almost a certainty. And if you are an addict, you can find refuge in Christ—that is an absolute certainty.

Day 6
Foxholes

Researchers who analyzed church attendance in the wake of the 9/11 attacks noted a spike in attendance directly following the tragedy. One megachurch in Dallas saw their attendance jump from 13,000 on September 9 to 21,000 on September 16. It was a time of unprecedented openness to God's leading, of individuals searching for stability and answers. Unfortunately, the mood soon passed.

This is what is known as the "foxhole faith syndrome." When the heat is on and the shells are whizzing overhead, we suddenly seek God.

We take on the attitude of David, who wrote, "Whoever dwells in the shelter of the Most High will rest in the shadow of the Almighty. I will say to the Lord, 'He is my refuge and my fortress, my God, in whom I trust'" (Psalm 91:1-2).

Most addicts turn to God because of a crisis. Then, when the crisis passes, so does their desire for God. But it doesn't have to be that way.

While serving in the Obama Administration, Rahm Emanuel famously said, "Never let a serious crisis go to waste. It's an opportunity to do things you didn't think you could do before."

Plug in the word "sobriety" in place of "things." You may be in a crisis time, seeking God in a foxhole you didn't know existed a few days ago. It's okay to be in a crisis. What's not okay is to let it go to waste.

Day 7
Worse than Failure

Sometimes, the only thing worse than a bad decision is a no-decision. Aaron Burr said, "Error is better than indecision."

King Rehoboam suffered from paralysis by analysis. He recoiled in the big moments. The king had the authority and power to meet every challenge successfully. But, crippled by his unwillingness to make decisions, he found himself in constant turmoil.

One day, the Bible says, "Some worthless scoundrels gathered around him and opposed Rehoboam, son of Solomon, when he was young and indecisive and not strong enough to resist them" (2 Chronicles 13:7).

Like Rehoboam, you have the authority and power to overcome. You have what it takes and you have Who it takes. Your recovery will be driven by making the decisions God clearly puts before you.

When you fail, it is more likely due to indecision than lack of knowledge. John Ortberg was right: "Greatness is never achieved through indecision."

Because he wouldn't make decisions, Rehoboam was "not strong enough to resist" the battles that came his way. Recovery only comes through the strength to resist, and the strength to resist only comes by making the decisions that are right in front of you.

Week 9
Secrets

"If you have to sneak to do it, lie to cover it up, or delete it to avoid it being seen, then you probably shouldn't be doing it."

- Bishop Dale Bronner

THIS WEEK'S EXERCISE
Get the Secrets Out

You are only as healthy as your secrets. They are who you really are. What you are when no one is looking is who you really are.

I'm sure there are other ways to say the same thing, but you get the point. It is what you are holding onto, what you haven't told anybody, that is holding you back. You must get the secrets out. You don't need to tell everybody, but you do need to tell somebody. Why? Because God can only *heal* what you *reveal*.

This exercise consists of three parts.

Part A—Identify your secret. Write it here: _____

_____

Part B—Decide who to tell: _____

Part C—Tell them. When will you tell them? _____

Day 1
Secrets

Secrets kill.

There is a story about a man named Achan. He cost Israel 36 lives and a huge upset loss to the army of tiny Ai. Israel had just defeated mighty Jericho. But they soon learned that yesterday's success is no guarantee of tomorrow's victory. They became overconfident and they lost. Worse yet, Achan broke God's command by keeping a few valuables from the previous battle. He confessed, "I coveted the silver and gold and buried them under my tent" (Joshua 7:21). And what he buried became his undoing. It would cost him his life.

Secrets kill.

The danger of our secrets is that they define us, whether we know it or not. French novelist André Malraux wrote, "Man is not what he thinks he is; he is what he hides."

Secrets kill.

Patrick Kennedy says, "No one is immune from addiction; it afflicts people of all ages, races, classes, and professions." If anyone should have been immune to addiction, it should have been Patrick Kennedy. But what he saw alcohol do to so many in his family, it did to him. And he did not find sobriety until he exposed his struggle to those around him. It took Kennedy years to learn this, but when he did, it saved his life. Patrick Kennedy learned this . . .

Secrets kill.

What are you hiding today? The only way you can kill the enemy is to expose it. Get it out into the open. Tell somebody. Today. Because secrets kill.

Day 2
The Fertilizer of Addiction

Secrecy is the fertilizer of addiction. Secrets kill everything in their sight—sobriety, recovery, and relationships. Edward Teller said it well: "Secrecy, once accepted, becomes an addiction."

German philosopher Georg Simmel added, "Every relationship between two individuals or two groups will be characterized by the ratio of secrecy that is involved in it."

You don't need to tell your secrets to *everyone*, but you do need to tell them to *someone*. Until you are known, you will not be well.

Think of it like this. You have a severe pain in your body, so you go see the doctor. He asks you how you injured yourself and where it hurts. You decide that is a secret not worth sharing. The doctor responds predictably. "If you aren't willing to tell me what happened and where it hurts, I can't help you."

Those who experience successful recovery have learned to tell others how they injured themselves and where it hurts.

I suggest you start by sharing the details with the God of whom Scripture says, "No one is hidden from his sight, but all are naked and exposed to the eyes of him to whom we must give an account" (Hebrews 4:13).

Day 3
Mulch

I have taken on a new project at our house. I care for the flower bed in front on the house. This means dealing with Satan's gift to horticulture—weeds.

About a week ago, as I was tending the plants, I saw one tiny weed in the back, approachable only on bended knee. I had to select my plan of action from among three options. I could crawl to the protected area and pull the weed by its roots. I could grab the top of the weed and remove the part my wife might see the next day. Or I could do the easy thing—toss a little mulch on the weed.

I chose option three. And it worked for a few days. Then the weed pointed its disgusting little head through my mulch. So I tossed more mulch. Eventually, I came to two conclusions: (1) I don't own enough mulch to win this battle, and (2) the only permanent solution was to pull the devil out by its roots.

Perhaps you've treated your sin like that weed. You covered it over with a little lie or alternative behaviors, and then pretended the problem no one could see must therefore not really exist. Then the activity returned, and it was worse. You kept treating the appearances until it happened—you ran out of mulch.

Eventually, you have to dig down where no one else can see and deal with the root. You will probably find trauma, abuse, and isolation there. It won't be an easy thing to do, but it's the only thing to do. There is no other way you will ever remove the sin that "so easily sets us back" (Hebrews 11:1).

Day 4
Possibilities

That great theologian Billy Joel said, "I'd rather laugh with the sinners than cry with the saints."

There is something to be said for laughing—even from the valley of addiction. Keeping things bottled up always makes things worse. But to whom do we turn? Whom do we tell? I know this. You better find that person, because keeping your struggle to yourself only leads to implosion from within.

Following his sin with Bathsheba, King David went through a period of cover-ups. He hid his sin, and to make matters worse, he had Bathsheba's husband put to death in order to have her for himself. It was all a part of a master plan to cover up what he had done.

And that worked—until it didn't. David would soon acknowledge, "When I kept silent my bones roared" (Psalm 32:3). He was saying, "Until I confessed what I had done to God and one other person, the pain shot down to my bones."

Secrets make us sick.

Dr. Alex Lickerman wrote, in *Psychology Today*, "Confession opens up possibilities we would otherwise miss."

What possibilities are you missing because of your secrets? A closer walk with God? A real connection with another human being? It's time to get it out. Tell someone. Then get ready to see possibilities you would otherwise surely miss.

Day 5
The Experience of Secrecy

Secrecy. I've experienced it, and it's not good.

Dr. Michael Slepian, professor at Columbia Business School and author of the study, *The Experience of Secrecy*, concludes, "The hardest thing about secrets isn't holding them, but living with them and thinking about them."

Ruben Castaneda wrote an article for U.S. News, titled *How Your Secrets Can Damage and Maybe Even Kill You*. He concluded, "You may be experiencing negative health effects from thinking about your secrets."

Dr. Jay Stringer says, "When we don't tell our secrets, our actions eventually will."

Jesus warned, "Nothing is covered up that will not be revealed, or hidden that will not be known" (Luke 12:2).

Here's the deal. Holding secrets does not equate to a life of addiction. But holding secrets precipitates a life of addiction. The solution? No more secrets.

Day 6
Shadows

Addiction thrives in the darkness.

Psychiatrist Carl Jung refers to our problem as a "shadow." The shadow is a metaphor for everything about us that we hide. We take our junk and hide it, repress it, deny it, and stuff it. We don't want anyone to see what's really going on inside of us. But there's just one problem.

Addiction thrives in the darkness.

In his marvelous book, *No More Secrets*, Dennis Swanberg writes, "If we cannot get rid of our secret, we try to get rid of ourselves by doing something that numbs us, amuses us, or makes us forget who we are." This only makes the problem worse.

Addiction thrives in the darkness.

There are 196 references and warnings in Scripture—about darkness. The psalmist wrote, "They do not know nor do they understand; they walk about in darkness. All the foundations of the earth are shaken" (Psalm 82:5). Our only hope of redemption is to step into the light, to be known, to embrace our better future. We must come out from the shadows. Why?

Addiction thrives in the darkness.

You must be known, not by everybody, but by somebody. Decide today to take that leap and share your story with someone you can trust. You must do this, because addiction thrives in the darkness.

Day 7
No More Secrets

George Orwell said, "If you want to keep a secret, you must hide it from your-self."

Isaiah 29:15 reads, "Woe to those who go to great depths to hide their plans from the Lord, who do their work in darkness and think, 'Who sees us? Who will know?'"

Dr. Michael Slepian wrote a paper in *Journal of Personality and Social Psychology*. Slepian said of secrets: "One problem with keeping secrets is that your goal becomes keeping secrets. Then your motivational system is centered on fulfilling this goal, which fixes your mind on that which has become your secret, and this leads to relapse. You keep thinking about the secret you are trying to protect."

Even your darkest, most intimate secrets must come to light. Why? Because secrets kill.

It is critical to get your secrets out. In 12-Step work, this is called "working the First Step." You must let go of your secrets—because secrets kill.

Week 10
Church

"Anyone who is to find Christ must first find the church. How could anyone know where Christ is and what faith is in him unless he knew where his believers are?"

- Martin Luther

THIS WEEK'S EXERCISE
Bless Your Church

As a senior pastor for 31 years, I learned that people join a church for only two reasons: (a) what they can get out of that church, and (b) what they can contribute to that church. And I rarely met anyone in the second group.

We generally pick a church based on how much we like the pastor, preaching, worship, small group, or some specific program that meets our individual needs. But church is like recovery. You get out of it only what you put into it.

Your exercise this week will be to give back to your church. Bless them in some way. I will offer several suggestions on how you might do this. Pick one of the following ideas, or come up with your own. Then record your feelings and reflections below.

Option #1—Write a letter of encouragement to your pastor.

Option #2—Make a financial donation to your church (above your regular gifts).

Option #3—Support an activity or group with your attendance.

Option #4—Visit a church member in the hospital or nursing home.

Option #5—Offer to serve one week as a greeter.

Option #6—Bring a friend to your church this week.

Personal reflections on how it felt and what it meant to serve your church:

_____

_____

_____

_____

_____

_____

Day 1
Lesson from Camden Yards

It was on my bucket list. A lover of the traditions of baseball, I had wanted to visit Baltimore's Camden Yards since the ballpark opened in 1992. In Baltimore for a meeting, I had one day to take in the significant sites of the Baltimore/Washington, D.C. area. I narrowed my options to the Lincoln Memorial, the White House, and Camden Yards. In choosing baseball over politics, I was reminded of the Babe Ruth quote of the 1920s. When asked to defend the fact that his salary eclipsed that of President Calvin Coolidge, Ruth explained, "I'm having a better year than he is."

The lessons from baseball to recovery are infinite. Let me cite one.

Baseball is a team sport.

The great Nolan Ryan once posted an ERA below 2.00—and had a losing record. "How was this possible?" he was asked. "It's simple," said Ryan. "I'm not a very good hitter."

Even Nolan Ryan could not win unless others on the team scored some runs. In recovery, you cannot make it by yourself. And this is the point where I see many addicts fail. You need a group, a sponsor, and accountability. You need a team.

Jesus prayed that we would be one (John 17:21). Why? Because he knew that we cannot make it without a team.

Babe Ruth and Nolan Ryan needed a team. So do you.

Day 2
What You Can't Do Without

You can *find* sobriety without community. But you can't *keep* sobriety without community. That is one reason God invented this thing we call the church.

Many have abandoned the church because they have been injured there. But if you have been hurt by a church, the answer isn't to abandon the whole idea, but to simply find another church.

Unless you know something God doesn't.

The Bible is clear. Hebrews 10:24-25 reads, "Let us consider how we may spur one another on toward love and good deeds, not giving up meeting together, as some are in the habit of doing, but encouraging one another—and all the more as you see the day approaching."

Jay Lowder, founder of Jay Lowder Harvest Ministries, writes, "People need the church to help them grow and mature. They also need the community of others who have the same passions and experiences. These relationships feed off of one another to help encourage, challenge, and grow one another. So no, you don't have to go to church to have a relationship with Jesus, but you do need to go to church if you're serious about making it stronger."

Tertullian said, "The blood of the martyrs is the seed of the church." That starts with Jesus. He gave his life for the church. And if the church mattered that much to God, it should matter to you.

There's no soft way to say this. Unless you are in a church, you are living outside the boundaries of God's Word. But the good news is that you can do something about it—starting this Sunday.

Day 3
Porn in the Pew

Josh McDowell said, "Porn is the greatest threat to the church in the history of the world."

So how serious is the porn problem in today's church? Let me quote a few statistics that I cite in my book, *Porn in the Pew*.

- 62% of men in church view porn monthly.
- 37% of pastors view porn.
- 29% of Christians believe porn is okay.
- 57% of pastors say porn is their church's #1 problem.
- Only 7% of churches offer any help for porn addicts.

Stuart Vogelman, executive director of *Pure Warriors Ministry*, says, "The church is going to have to decide if it's going to fight to be the pure bride of Christ. It's probably going to be the toughest battle the church has ever faced, and most churches are not equipped for it."

So how can the church respond to the porn epidemic? I suggest the following:

- Recognize the magnitude of the problem.
- Appoint and train an addiction ministry leader.
- Create a culture of redemption.
- Start men's and women's groups.

- Host 12-Step groups.
- Sponsor annual events.
- Provide addiction counseling.
- Use **There's Still Hope** as a resource!

Paul warned, "Let us cleanse ourselves from all filthiness of the flesh and spirit, perfecting holiness in the fear of the Lord" (2 Corinthians 7:1). Josh McDowell is right. Porn is the major threat to the church today. We must respond now. *You must respond now!*

Day 4
A United Front

A man was rescued from a deserted island, where he had lived since his boat went off track ten years earlier. His rescuers noticed that he had built three structures on the island. They asked him why he built each hut.

The man replied, "Well, that first hut over there—that's where I live. The second hut is where I go to church. And the third hut is where I used to go to church."

Christians are not known for getting along with each other. But Paul pleaded, "I appeal to you, brothers and sisters, in the name of our Lord Jesus Christ, that all of you agree with one another in what you say and that there be no divisions among you, but that you be perfectly united in mind and thought" (1 Corinthians 1:10).

C.S. Lewis described the way the Body of Christ is intended to operate. "True friends face in the same direction, toward common projects, interests, and goals."

The fight against porn and sex addiction must be engaged by a unified front. If we as Christ-followers won't stand for this, we'll fall for anything.

Day 5
The Effects of Isolation

In November of 2018, a professional poker player bet on himself. Rich Alati bet $100,000 that he could live in total darkness for 30 days. He lost.

Alati was placed in a small room, completely dark. He had a bed, fridge, food, water, and bathroom—all the physical necessities of life. But he couldn't make it past 20 days. The changes in his sleep cycle, repeated bouts with hallucinations, and abject loneliness overcame him.

Isolation is a deadly condition. One of the reasons living in isolation is difficult is that humans are social creatures. Many who live in isolated environments—such as researchers in Antarctica—report that loneliness is the most difficult part of their job. They often become overcome with depression and fail to process simple information. When living in darkness, the effects of isolation become even more magnified.

This is a parable on life. Isolation drives many men and women into addiction. Isolation will take you further than you want to go, keep you longer than you want to stay, and cost you more than you want to pay.

That's why the early followers of Christ "devoted themselves to the apostles' teaching *and to the fellowship*, to the breaking of bread and the prayers" (Acts 2:42).

Quit isolating. Let me suggest three ways: (a) join a small group at church, (b) get into a 12-Step meeting, and (c) become accountable to one other person.

Day 6
The Best Sermon

Orel Hershiser was having a bad day. The future all-star pitcher was laboring on the mound when his manager, Tommy Lasorda, left the dugout for a brief visit. Lasorda got in Hershiser's face and proceeded to tell him what he could become as a pitcher. "You're a winner!" Lasorda said. After the manager returned to the dugout, Hershiser struck out the side.

The pitcher looks back on that as a turning point in his career. He credits Lasorda for what he calls the "Sermon on the Mound."

We all need to hear a good sermon from time to time. But the best sermon is not preached in the pulpit as often as it is in the office, on the golf course, or in the mirror.

Yes—in the mirror.

Jerry Bridges, author of *The Pursuit of Happiness*, wisely wrote, "Preach to yourself daily."

The prophet declared, "The righteousness of the righteous shall be upon himself" (Ezekiel 18:20). In other words, we must own our recovery. And we must be our own best encourager.

We all need to hear an encouraging "Sermon on the Mound." If you know someone who is down, visit their mound. But in the meantime, be your own congregation. Remind yourself daily: you're still in the game, God is on your team, and your team will eventually win.

Be encouraged today, if not by someone else, then by yourself.

Day 7
Dance Partners

It was the deadliest dance of all time.

In the ancient city of Strasbourg, in modern-day France, hundreds of citizens broke out in dance one day in 1518. But for some reason, they did not stop. They danced for hours, and then days. Dozens died from exhaustion. While history provides no clear answer as to why they didn't stop dancing before it killed them, one thing is certain.

Each dancer did what the other dancers were doing.

Paul warned, "Bad company corrupts good character" (1 Corinthians 15:33).

St. Augustine offered great wisdom on the subject. "Bad company is like a nail driven into a post, which, after the first and second blow, may be drawn out with little difficulty; but being once driven up to the head, the pincers cannot take hold to draw it out, but which can only be done by the destruction of the wood."

Let me translate: be careful in choosing your dance partner.

If you are to walk in the right direction, it will occasionally require that you walk away from the crowd. Be careful in picking your dance partners.

Week 11
3-Second Rule

"I made a covenant with my eyes to not look lustfully at a young woman."

- Job 31:1

THIS WEEK'S EXERCISE
Get a Rubber Band

As a sex addict, your brain has been conditioned neurologically to your acting out behaviors. Many sex addicts were exposed to pornography at a young age and began to masturbate and/or fantasize about it. Every time the addict ejaculated, he sent a rush of chemicals to his brain called endorphins and enkephalins. The brain, as an organ of the body, has no morality. It just knows when it receives a rush of pleasure-inducing chemicals. This feels good. The rush could be from heroin, sky diving, sex, or cocaine. Regardless of what caused the rush, the brain, as an organ, would not have a moral dilemma on how it received this rush.

After frequent ejaculations brought on by acting out, the sex addict begins to develop neurological pathways in the brain while acting out sexually. The brain, as an organ, adjusts to getting its neurological need met by the cycle of going into a fantasy state and minutes later sending the brain a rush of chemicals through ejaculation.

To recover from sexual addiction, you must retrain your brain to not connect the fantasy world with these moments of release and relief. To stop this biological cycle that you have had in place for years, you will need a biological reconditioning cycle. One way to facilitate this is today's simple exercise.

Place a rubber band on either wrist, and when you start to have sexually inappropriate thoughts, snap the rubber band on the inside of your wrist. This sets up a cycle in your brain that says "fantasy = pain" instead of "fantasy = pleasure." The body is designed to avoid pain, so this will reduce the amount of fantasies you are having and eventually lessen the inappropriate thoughts, so you can focus on your freedom. You can memorize and quote helpful Scriptures to strengthen your spirit when you snap the rubber band, but use this rubber band to recondition your brain.

According to Dr. Doug Weiss, the person who commits to this reconditioning exercise of the brain finds that about 80% of the fantasy lifestyle subsides within about 30 days. It continues throughout the first 90 days. This is a helpful exercise to "take your thoughts captive."

The date I placed the rubber band on my wrist:_____

The date I removed the rubber band: _____

Day 1
The Eyes Have It

Job knew what it was to live a disciplined life. Late in his story, we read this: "I made a covenant with my eyes, that I would not sin against God" (Job 31:1).

That was a smart move, as the Bible warns against the "lust of the eyes" (1 John 2:26).

You need to learn to control your eyes for the sake of your sobriety, but also if you love your wife. When you look at other women, you are telling your wife three things: (a) you are selfish, (b) you lack self-control, and (c) you are probably even worse when your wife isn't with you.

Steve Harvey said, "A woman can't change a man because she loves him. A man changes himself because he loves her."

Here's my advice. Learn the 3-second rule. It's simple. This practice dictates that when you see an attractive person, you never allow yourself to look beyond three seconds. It is similar to what Stephen Arterburn calls "bouncing the eyes." But I put a time limit on it, so you can define "bouncing." When you see someone attractive, count to three—quickly. And make sure you have looked away before you get to 3.

Do what Job did. Make a covenant with your eyes.

Day 2
A Fish Bowl

Imagine I am setting an empty fish bowl in front of you. That bowl represents a person's brain. Then, one by one, I drop several golf balls into the bowl, until it can't hold any more. These balls represent different thoughts housed in your brain. Then I ask you if the bowl appears full. "Yes," you say dutifully.

"Not so quick," I respond. Then imagine that I reach for a pitcher of water and slowly begin pouring the water into the fish bowl.

Here's the lesson. When it seems the bowl is full, it really isn't. And that water will eventually touch every part of the "brain."

The water represents porn. Your brain appears to be full of thoughts, memories, emotions, and information. But there is always room for one more image. And when you take these images in, they corrupt the rest of your brain.

The Bible says, "A little yeast leavens the whole batch of dough" (Galatians 5:9).

You may think your brain is full. But it always has room for more images that will rewire everything. So be careful. Be on alert.

Protect your brain from every stray image.

Day 3
Lessons from Golf

I am to golf what rap is to music. Technically, I am a golfer, as I have hacked at the ball an average of once a year over the past ten years. One day I was playing out of the rough. There was a tree directly between me and the green. God knew my ball would be right there, but he stuck a tree in my path anyway. I never hit my target, so I aimed right for the tree. Then it hit me—the ball, that is. It didn't hit the trunk of the tree, just a small branch. But that was enough. It turned a promising double bogey into something far worse.

Bobby Jones was right when he said, "Golf is the closest game to the game we call life."

I'm not sure Jones would have said that had he seen me play. But there is a lesson, for sure. Be careful what you are aiming at, because you just might hit it.

I know guys who mess around on their phones, browsing dating sites and soft-porn sites. They never intend to actually line up a meeting with a woman, nor do they plan to click on the porn sites. But inevitably, they do. Why? Because what we aim at, we hit. And then it hits us.

Paul warned the church, "Whoever sows to please their flesh, from the flesh will reap destruction; whoever sows to please the Spirit, from the Spirit will reap eternal life" (Galatians 6:8).

Whatever captures your eye today will own your heart tomorrow. So be careful where you look—in golf and in life.

Make a covenant with your eyes, to only look at those things that feed your spirit and starve your addiction.

Day 4
Involuntary Slavery

"Jesus said, 'Very truly I tell you, everyone who sins is a slave to sin'" (John 8:34).

Ancient philosophy taught that those who are devoted to their lusts are subject to the most degrading kind of slavery. You own your addiction, then your addiction owns you.

The word Jesus used for "slave" was *doulos*. It refers to an involuntary state. We do not volunteer to become slaves to our addictions. The physiology of sex addiction confirms this.

After the sex act, addicts quickly slide into despair, their dopamine receptors left hungry for more sex. This craving is set up biologically and physiologically. Quick fixes provide a state of ecstasy and nirvana. But it doesn't last. The addict is rendered emptier, distressed, and fragmented. To quell these painful feelings, he is compelled to resume his pursuit of the next fix.

In the SA (Sexaholics Anonymous) White Book, it says, "The only way we knew to be free of it was to do it."

John Calvin nailed it when he said, "Men are destitute of freedom unless they find it in Christ."

Addicts are slaves to their drug of choice. For the sex addict, this leads him or her down a cruel journey of isolation and despair. That is why successful recovery is a spiritual recovery. It cannot be done apart from the One who sets us free.

Day 5
Just a Flesh Wound

In *Monty Python and the Holy Grail*, the Black Knight (John Cleese) told King Arthur (Graham Chapman), after losing both arms in combat, "It's just a flesh wound."

That is the picture of every addict in denial. We've all said it—"It's not that bad." "It's just porn." "It was just a one-time thing." *"It's just a flesh wound."*

Minimizing is the art of the delusional. What other choice do we really have? In our addiction, we can either say, "Yes, I am a sex addict" (which calls for radical change) or we can minimize.

Pamela Nikodem writes, "Minimization is a side-step away from denial of any personal responsibility in a situation or incident."

In what ways do we minimize our disease? Here are a few of the examples I hear from clients:

1. Looks and glances
2. Fantasy

3. Euphoric recall
4. Missed 12-Step meetings
5. Lax recovery work

The answer is to respond to every misstep with immediate correction. It is better to overreact than underreact. There are no minor setbacks. And every time you minimize something, all you're really doing is making it bigger.

Day 6
Tape Recorder vs. Camera

Your brain is not a tape recorder. It's a camera. Let me explain.

Try to remember the first person you were sexually attracted to. Now think of the first person you kissed. Finally, think of the first provocative picture, image, or poster you saw.

That was the easy part.

Now, think of a single lecture from grades 1-12.

That was the hard part.

You remember the images because your brain is a camera. If it was a tape recorder, you would have remembered at least one of the 12,000 classroom lectures you sat through by the time you graduated from high school.

Now, this is a problem. When you drink in an image of pornography, well, I have bad news. You can try to overcome that image by thinking about rainbows, flowers, and a deer in your front yard. But the sex images just won't go away. These images can be managed, but not erased.

The solution? Determine, from this day forward, to not take in any of these images. The Bible offers a better plan when it says to focus on "the wife of your youth" (Ecclesiastes 9:9).

Day 7
Collect Calls

2 Corinthians 10:5 tells us to "take captive every thought to make it obedient to Christ."

Let me once again emphasize the "3-second rule." When your eyes are triggered or an intrusive thought or memory invades your mind, move away from it within three seconds. Then say a prayer, read a verse, make a call.

Focus on that last one—make a call.

Back in the day, we had this thing in our house we called a land line. It was a precursor to the modern cell phone. We called it a telephone. When someone wanted to contact us, they dialed our number, and this thing would ring. We'd pick up the receiver. And sometimes, it would be what we called a "long distance call." This one cost money. We'd hear the voice of the "operator," who would ask us if we were willing to "accept" a call that was made "collect." In other words, once we knew who was trying to call us, we had about three seconds to decide if we were willing to pay to hear what they had to say.

Lustful thoughts make collect calls. They will enter our minds from time to time. That is reality. It's what we do with those thoughts that matters. When we accept the call, it will cost us—mightily.

Aristotle said it like this. "It is the mark of an educated mind to be able to entertain a thought without accepting it."

Temptations always call collect. You will recognize the voice. And when you do, don't negotiate the price or ask what he/she wants. Just hang up—fast!

Week 12
End Game

*"We cannot go back and create a whole new beginning,
but we can begin now, and make a whole new ending."*

- Carl Bard

THIS WEEK'S EXERCISE
Predict the End Game

Addiction always does three things: (a) it takes you further than you want to go, (b) it keeps you longer than you want to stay, and (c) it costs you more than you want to pay. It never ends well. You must end the carnage before the carnage ends you. You know this addiction has robbed you of joy, peace, relationships, and much more. But here's the scary part . . .

It could actually get worse.

Until we hit bottom, we rarely bounce up. So what would your bottom look like? Let's predict the end game. If you don't stay sober and live in permanent recovery, how will life look in five years? How will things end for you?

Sometimes, fear is a great motivator. When you are tempted to act out, refer to this exercise, because you are about to write down what your life will look like in five years if you don't get help soon.

Describe the end game below. If you continue to act out, what will your life look like in five years?

Your family life: _____

_____

_____

_____

Your spiritual life: _____

_____

_____

_____

Your physical life: _____

_____

_____

_____

Your financial life: _____

_____

_____

_____

Other: _____

_____

_____

_____

Day 1
Famous Last Words

"Pardon me, sir. I meant not to do it."

Those were the last words of Marie Antoinette. At the height of the French revolution, Louis XVI of France and his wife Marie Antoinette were charged with treason and sent to the guillotine. After a humiliating ride through the streets of Paris, she was brought to the guillotine. While on the scaffold, Marie accidentally stepped on her executioner's foot and respectfully apologized, "Pardon me, sir. I meant not to do it." Seconds later, he chopped off her head.

Here are some other examples of famous last words. Beethoven: "Friends applaud, the comedy is finished." Humphrey Bogart: "I should have never switched from Scotch to Martinis." Winston Churchill: "I'm bored with it all." Frank Sinatra: "I'm losing it."

Drummer Buddy Rich died after surgery in 1987. As he was being prepped for surgery, his nurse asked him, "Is there anything you can't take?" Rich replied, "Yes, country music."

Paul's last recorded words were, "I have fought the good fight, I have finished the race, I have kept the faith" (2 Timothy 4:7).

Nothing in life matters more than finishing strong. Your addiction may have cost you your marriage, career, and reputation. But it need not define you. In order to have a better future, you have to quit trying to have a better past. It's time to move on. Make the rest count.

Fight the good fight. Finish the race. Keep the faith.

Day 2
Two-by-Fours

The Bible says, "Therefore love the Lord your God and keep his commands" (Deuteronomy 11:1).

What God said in the Old Testament still applies today. We are to follow his plan for our lives with consistency and persistency. The key to lasting recovery is hard work—repeated over time.

Albert Einstein shared the key to his success. "It's not that I'm so smart, it's just that I stay at it longer."

Recovery is all about staying at it.

A man walked into a lumber yard and asked for some two-by-fours. The merchant wanted to make sure he cut the wood according to the customer's specifications, so he said, "Okay, two-by-fours. We can do that. But how long do you want them?"

The customer said, "A long time. I'm using them to build a house."

You need to put in place a recovery plan that will last for a long time. If you want your recovery to last, build it with enduring materials: go to meetings, pray the Serenity Prayer every day, and stay connected to others on the same path.

Do things that make recovery last. It starts with obeying God's commands—over and over, day after day.

Day 3
Don't Quit Now!

One of the keys to successful recovery is the determination to never give up, even in the face of slips and relapse. We only lose when we quit fighting.

No one personified this spirit better than Abraham Lincoln. He knew failure first-hand. In 1816 his family was forced out of their home. Two years later, his mother died. In 1831 he failed in business. The next year, he ran for the Illinois state legislature and lost. He lost his job as well. In 1833 he borrowed money to live on and needed 17 years to pay it back. In 1835 his fiancée died. This led to a nervous breakdown that had Lincoln in bed for six months. He would lose races for Congress, the Senate, and Vice President before being elected President of the United States.

Reflecting on his losses, Lincoln said, "The path was worn and slippery. My foot slipped from under me, but I said, 'It's only a slip, not a fall.'"

We must see our failures as slips and not falls. The key is to keep at it. Recovery is a marathon, not a sprint.

I love the Book of Nehemiah. When called back to his homeland to lead the rebuilding of the wall around Jerusalem, Nehemiah faced a prodigious task. But with the help of God and those closest to him, he prevailed.

What worked for Nehemiah will work for you. "We rebuilt the wall till all of it reached half its height, for the people worked with all their heart" (Nehemiah 4:6).

When progress comes slowly, keep at it. Recovery will come, if, like the people on Nehemiah's team, you "work with all your heart."

Day 4
The Best Is Yet to Come

"I've lost everything."

The call from a man I had never met had a familiar message. A good man, successful by all measures, had served his churches with distinction. "Bob" had been a senior pastor for over 30 years. But now he had lost it all—his church, his ministry, and even his wife. His porn habit had been discovered. I recognized true remorse and repentance in his voice—and loss.

What do you tell a man like Bob? You tell him to read the Book of Job. If anyone could relate to losing everything, it was Job. He literally lost the farm, and worse yet, his family.

We are all too familiar with how the Book of Job begins. But we forget how it ends.

"The Lord blessed the latter part of Job's life more than the former part. He had 14,000 sheep, 6,000 camels, 1,000 yoke of oxen, and 1,000 donkeys" (Job 42:12).

Did you catch that? "The Lord blessed the latter part of Job's life more than the former part."

Dale Carnegie observed, "Most of the important things in the world have been accomplished by people who have kept on trying when there seemed to be no hope at all."

For Bob there is hope. For you there is hope. Even if you've lost everything, the Lord can bless the latter part of your life more than the former part.

Have you lost everything? Take heart, for we have a God who can do in your future more than he had done in your past. The best is yet to come.

Day 5
Getting Past the Past

We all know the tragedy that became the life of Job. We remember him as a man of unspeakable loss and pain. When his life was shattered by one disaster after another, Job and his counselor friends wrestled with this question: "How do we explain such suffering?"

But there's more to the story.

Only in the last five chapters of the Book do we find God finally joining the conversation. And does he ever! God fires more than 60 questions at the tongue-tied Job. The gist of these queries seems to be, "I don't have to explain myself to you. I am the Creator and you are my creature."

Job responded well: "I know that you can do anything and no plan of yours can be thwarted" (42:2).

And then the blessings flowed. God gave Job more in the last part of his life than he ever had in the beginning.

Pastor Bayless Conley said, "These verses declare that there are only two things you need in order to succeed. First, you must be convinced that God can turn anything into glory. Second, you must be completely convinced and persuaded that God loves you unconditionally."

Here's the lesson. Mistakes, tragedy, and suffering are all a part of God's bigger plan. Failure and missteps are an integral part of God's design for your life. Don't regret them; embrace them. Never forget this timeless truth—what God has allowed in your past, he will use in your future.

Whether your suffering has been self-induced or not, leave it in the past. Let God use it to create a future you could otherwise never know.

Day 6
Happy Endings

I love the story of the little boy whose mother took him to the animal shelter to pick out a dog. He chose the homeliest looking puppy, but one whose tail was wagging briskly. His mom asked the boy why he picked that particular dog. The boy said, "I wanted the dog with a happy ending."

We all like happy endings.

Here's the good news. We win. For those whose faith is in their Higher Power, there is coming a day when "He will wipe every tear from their eyes. There will be no more death, no more tears, no more sorrow, and no more pain" (Revelation 21:4).

You may be in a battle today—for custody of your eyes, purity of thought, and sobriety. And while you may not win every battle, you will win the war. Your story has a happy ending.

Robin Sharma, Canadian writer and speaker, says, "Starting strong is good. Finishing strong is epic."

Billy Sunday offered a baseball analogy. "Stopping at third adds no more to the score than striking out. It doesn't matter how well you start if you fail to finish."

Keep your eye on the prize. There is coming a day when you will be victorious. The road ahead will be marred by potholes, occasional detours, and moments of discouragement. But I've read the end of the Book. There is a happy ending.

Take a moment today to reflect on the fact that by faith in God, your journey will end well. There will be a happy ending. For that you can be thankful.

Day 7
End Game

You are going to die. But don't feel singled out. That applies to pretty much everyone.

Jesus said, "You must be ready, because the Son of Man will come at an hour when you do not expect him" (Luke 12:40).

Elton Trueblood said, "Our life is a gift from God. What we do with that life is our gift to God."

What have you done with your life? If you had just one week to live, how would you spend it? Would you try to fulfill a lifelong dream? Would you make sure you said your good-byes to loved ones? Or would you indulge in all kinds of pleasures, expecting to make your life right with God in some sort of "deathbed conversion" at the last possible moment?

I just read an article by Kimberly Hiss titled, *16 Things Smart People Do to Prepare for Death*.

Amos had only one: "Prepare to meet thy God" (Amos 4:12).

I'm with Amos on this one. We need to keep it simple. Prepare to meet God. Let that inform every decision you make about recovery.

Prepare to meet God because it could happen at any moment. I'd tell you what that means about your acting out, but I'm pretty sure you already know.

Week 13
Inner Circle

"In the inner circle, we put the sexual behaviors we want to abstain from. These are the behaviors that we identify as addictive, harmful, or unacceptable to us."

- AA Three Circles Worksheet

THIS WEEK'S EXERCISE
Identify Your Inner Circle

Your inner circle behaviors are those activities that reverse your sobriety. Most of these activities will be obvious. If you aren't sure which activities belong in your inner circle, consult with your spouse, therapist, or sponsor. While some people might place some of the examples below in their middle circle (rather than inner circle), it is best to err on the side of safety. I suggest you define your inner circle behaviors as follows:

- Sex with myself or any other person other than my spouse
- Anything that will almost always lead me to receive sexual stimulation (act out)

Check the activities that you will place in your inner circle. Add to this list, as needed.

- Sexual contact with another person (other than my spouse) _____
- Masturbation _____
- Viewing of pornography _____
- Browsing dating sites _____
- Browsing social media _____
- Contacting a former acting out partner _____
- Visiting sexually oriented businesses _____
- Other: _____
- Other: _____
- Other: _____
- Other: _____
- Other: _____

Day 1
Must I Hit Rock Bottom?

I am often asked, "Do I really need to hit bottom in order to find successful recovery?"

The therapists at Fairbanks Recovery offer this take. The presumption that one must "hit rock bottom" in order to get well is based on faulty reasoning. They write, "This myth is particularly troublesome because it packs a one-two punch. It propels the addict deeper into his addiction. And it causes family members to believe they are powerless to step in until someone has lost it all. But in reality, experts in addiction recovery can help addicts during any point in their journey. The sooner they get treatment, the more likely it is that they will recover and live a life free from their addiction."

Can someone get well before they hit bottom? Of course, they can! If we didn't believe that, we would be saying that God is powerless to heal a disease until it has worsened to its final phase.

We don't wait to pray for a cancer patient until her disease has reached Stage 4. We don't hold our prayers for someone with bronchitis until they have pneumonia. And we should pray for—and help—those in addiction the moment we learn of their disease.

Jesus said, "Come unto me all you who are burdened" (Matthew 11:28). His invitation is not closed to anyone.

Can someone find recovery before hitting rock bottom? Yes, they can. But only if they really want it.

Day 2
Clogged Arteries

I recently attended a church where the pastor told the following story. As a kid, he used to attend Houston Astros games with his dad. But on the long walk from the parking lot to their seats, his dad would often have to stop several times to catch his breath. Eventually, he went to the doctor, who diagnosed him with multiple clogged arteries. He was functioning on about 30 percent of his normal capacity.

The same is true for many of us. We have been walking along, functioning at less than our full capacity. The problem is that our hearts are clogged—by porn, fantasy, and infidelity.

Patrick F. Fagan, of the Family Research Council, produced a study on the effects of pornography on the heart. His 28-page report concluded that the use of porn results in "distorted attitudes and perceptions about the nature of the gift of sex."

In other words, porn clogs the arteries.

The Bible offers a special promise for those who keep their hearts free of porn and other forms of impurity. Jesus promised, "Blessed are the pure in heart, for they shall see God" (Matthew 5:8).

The man at the Astros game could barely walk because there was something wrong with his heart. The same is true in recovery. Until your heart is right, your walk won't be right.

Day 3
Is Sex a Need?

The reason many men use for acting out is that sex is a need, and they aren't "getting it" at home. But is that really true? Is sex a need?

In his article, *Sex and Our Psychological Needs*, Dr. Mark Manson answers this directly. He writes, "Psychologists have studied a number of psychological needs, but you can really narrow them down to four fundamental needs: (a) security, (b) self-esteem, (c) autonomy, and (d) connection."

Manson continues, "To be happy, stable people, we need to meet all four of these needs consistently. If not, our minds begin to rationalize ways to get them met. But here's the truth: sex is a strategy we use to meet our psychological needs and not a need itself."

We know this is true, because there is no evidence that celibacy leads to a psychologically unhealthy life.

What happens, Manson concludes, is that "people develop neuroses and addictions to get their needs met."

Here's the good news. If you aren't in a relationship that meets your sexual desires, remind yourself of this—they are desires, not needs. Your need is for (a) security, (b) self-esteem, (c) autonomy, and (d) connection. And those needs can be met by God.

Day 4
Death March

Memorize this truth—addiction will take you further than you want to go, keep you longer than you want to stay, and cost you more than you want to pay.

Solomon described the plight of the man who seeks a prostitute. "All at once he followed her like an ox going to the slaughter, like a deer stepping into a noose" (Proverbs 7:22).

It is a death march. We follow our passions blindly—into a trap. What starts as a moment of pleasure ends in a lifetime of shame. We lose our reputation, family, health, and minds. But we still do it. Such is the cunning and baffling nature of this disease.

Here's the process, as described by Thomas A. Kempis: "Sin is first a simple suggestion, then a strong imagination, then delight, then assent."

Satan tempted Adam with a suggestion. He tempted Jesus the same way. That's his M.O. Suggestion leads to imagination, which leads to brief pleasure. And then it's all over.

So what's the solution? It's simple. Don't negotiate with the enemy. By even entering into the discussion, you have gone too far. The rest is predictable. And sad.

Day 5
How to Stop Masturbation

Masturbation often leads to long-term depression, difficulty with a real sex life, loss of self-respect, and chronic fatigue. Therapist Betty Miller calls masturbation "one of Satan's devices." Masturbation is almost always accompanied by lust and fantasy. Adultery of the heart is a sin, according to Jesus (Matthew 5:28). I often hear from men who have become convinced that God desires for them to stop masturbation; I'm still waiting for a call from someone who says God actually led them to start masturbating.

So how do we stop masturbation in our personal lives? Let me offer a few suggestions.

1. Let go of self-condemnation. In order to have a better future, you must quit trying to have a better past. What's done is done. Forgive your past and move forward.

2. Remove all possible triggers. Start with access to porn and toxic relationships. Remove illicit channels from your television. Get on Covenant Eyes.
3. Create healthy outlets for time and energy. Stay busy. Engage a new hobby or fitness routine. Limit down time.
4. Stay in the game. If at first you don't succeed, you're normal. Don't give up. Alter your plan as needed.
5. See a therapist. I suggest seeing a Certified Sex Addiction Therapist (C.S.A.T.).

Masturbation is not your friend. But it is not a habit that will go away on its own. You must be proactive. Start with these five steps—one day at a time.

Day 6
Text & Drive

In 48 states, it is illegal to text and drive. (I won't divulge the other two states, but you might want to avoid driving through New Hampshire and Connecticut until further notice.) On an average day in America, nine citizens die in car wrecks caused by distracted driving. And while 90 percent of Americans agree that texting while driving is dangerous, 49% admit to still doing it.

So why do so many of us still text while driving? It's simple: (a) we think we can do both things at the same time, (b) we don't think we will get caught, and (c) we don't think anyone will get hurt.

The only thing more dangerous than texting and driving at the same time is doing porn and life at the same time. I know what you're thinking: (a) you can do both at the same time, (b) you won't get caught, and (c) no one will get hurt.

Well, guess what? You can't maintain a double life, you will get caught, and those you cherish most will pay a price for your reckless behavior. What you are doing is like a man texting while driving—with his family in the car. When he crashes, he's not the only one who gets hurt.

Solomon said, "You can't walk on coals and not get scorched" (Proverbs 6:27).

By using porn, you are walking on coals. You are playing with fire. Your reckless behavior is endangering those you love most. You need to pull over—while there's still time.

Day 7
Amazing Grace

The year was 1779. Anglican clergyman John Newton wrote *Amazing Grace* out of his personal experience. In 1748, a violent storm battered his ship off the coast of County Donegal, Ireland. Desperate for survival, Newton cried out to God. This marked his spiritual conversion. Looking back on that moment 31 years later, he penned what would become the signature hymn of the Second Great Awakening. To date, at least ten million recordings of Christianity's most famous hymn have been sold in over 100 languages.

Amazing Grace.

Grace is the sinner's best friend. Paul wrote, "Grace to you and peace from God our Father and the Lord Jesus Christ" (1 Corinthians 1:3). Paul was Exhibit A of grace. He didn't choose Christ; Christ chose him. It was grace that arrested Paul's attention on the road to Damascus. It was grace that spared Paul's life from a shipwreck. It was grace that freed him from prison. And it was grace that eventually welcomed him home—into the arms of the One whom he had proclaimed to Jews and Gentiles alike.

Have you hit bottom with your struggle with sexually compulsive behaviors? Have you stepped into a season of depression you didn't know existed? Have you discovered the unfaithfulness of your spouse?

Embrace grace. Philip Yancey nailed it: "Grace, like water, flows to the lowest part." If you find yourself "in the lowest part" today, cry out for grace. It will be your best friend.

Week 14
Sacrifice

"In order to provide for your breakfast of ham and eggs, the chicken made a donation, while the pig made a sacrifice."

\- Business Fable

THIS WEEK'S EXERCISE
Sacrifice this Week

When the disciples asked Jesus where they had fallen short, he told them that the greatest miracles come through prayer and fasting. It's that fasting thing that trips most of us up. We are okay with asking God to remove our compulsive tendencies. But fasting sounds a lot like sacrifice.

Recovery is a series of trade-offs. You have to give something to gain something. Sacrifice accomplishes two things: (a) it focuses you on what matters, and (b) it positions your heart to hear from, and respond to God.

Below are some examples of one act of sacrifice you might engage this week. Pick one, then reflect on the benefits you felt from making this sacrifice.

One act of sacrifice this week:

- Fasting one meal _____
- Making a financial donation to a recovery ministry _____
- Fasting from television for one day _____
- Spending time with someone who is new to recovery _____
- Volunteering to do something at my church _____
- Doing a random act of kindness for someone else _____
- Other: _____

Reflect on this act of sacrifice. How did it make you feel? How did this act of sacrifice affect your sobriety? Is this something you think you will do again in the future? How could you have made this sacrifice more wisely?

_____

_____

_____

Day 1
The Threshing Floor

God told King David to build an altar of sacrifice on the threshing floor of a man named Araunah. So David set out, money in pocket, ready to purchase the site of the altar as well as the animals that would be offered. Araunah was honored to help the king, so he offered both the site and the animals. David turned down the kind offer. He said, "I will not give God that which costs me nothing" (2 Samuel 24:24).

Many of us never learn the benefits of sacrifice.

In *Falling Upward*, Richard Rohr says, "The task of the first half of life is to build a self. The task of the second half of life is to lay that self down."

Sometimes, overcoming pornography is diminished to just that—laying it down. Every time you commit sexual sin, it is a choice. You may have the "Big 3" deep-seated in your background—trauma, abuse, and isolation. But still, every time you look at porn or commit any other sexual sin, it is a choice.

The answer is sacrifice. You must do two things: (a) lay yourself down before God, and (b) lay your habit down.

Repeat after me—"I will not give God that which costs me nothing."

Day 2
Mark Twain

Mark Twain said, "The best way to keep your health is to eat what you don't want, drink what you don't like, and do what you'd rather not."

The same is true in recovery from any addiction. It is self-indulgence that feeds the addiction, and self-sacrifice that paves the roadway out.

Jesus said it like this: "Whoever wants to save his life will lose it, but whoever loses his life for me will save it" (Luke 9:24).

Let's go back to what Mark Twain said. If I ate all I wanted, I'd weigh 400 pounds. If I drank all I wanted, I'd be the national spokesperson for Mountain Dew. And if I did all I wanted, I'd probably be divorced, living in shame, and broke.

Recovery, when you break it all down, comes down to one question—*Do you want the freedom from your habit more than the benefits that it provides?*

Answer that one right, and you're on your way out of the woods.

The only thing that is more difficult than recovery is addiction. You can find your way to freedom, but it's going to require sacrifice.

Day 3
Impossible!

One day in the late 1800s a religious leader was asked his opinion on the possibility of flight. "Nonsense!" he said. "We'll never fly!"

The name of the religious leader was Bishop Wright. The names of his two boys were Orville and Wilbur. Perhaps you've heard of them.

What seems impossible is often made possible.

An angel told Mary—still a virgin—that she would give birth to a really important son. When she questioned the plausibility of such an occurrence, the angel assured her, "Nothing shall be impossible with God" (Luke 1:37).

What seems impossible is often made possible.

I love the words of Lincoln Brewster's song, *God of the Impossible*. He wrote, "You are who you are—the God of the impossible."

What does this mean for recovery? Everything. When it seems there is no way you can maintain sobriety and find lasting recovery, pause and remember . . .

What seems impossible is often made possible.

Stop right now and say it with me. What seems impossible is often made possible.

Day 4
It's All About Pleasure

Why do men have extramarital affairs? Let me offer a simplistic response—pleasure. They do it for the pleasure of the moment.

But an affair is like a city holding a parade for winning a Super Bowl they had actually lost. When the parade is over, the reality sets in, as well as the pain. Cathy Meyer says it like this: "Extramarital affairs cause a ripple effect. The damage is always far more than you can see."

Still, men—and women—are entering into extramarital relationships at a record pace. Why? I'll say it again—pleasure. It's all based on the original "fake news." Somewhere along the line, we have come to believe that we were created for pleasure.

I agree with David Platt: "In a world that says, 'Promote, protect, and provide for yourself,' Jesus says, 'Crucify yourself.'"

Paul wrote, "For we know that our old self was crucified with him so that the body ruled by sin might be done away with, that we should no longer be slaves to sin" (Romans 6:6).

If you are in a relationship that violated your personal moral code, just be honest. Quit blaming your addiction, your spouse, your parents, or your horoscope. Admit it—you are choosing to live for pleasure rather than living for God. You have every opportunity to make that choice. Just own it.

Day 5
No Pain, No Gain

"No pain, no gain."

Ben Franklin is often credited as the originator of that famous line. In 1758, Ben became the Dave Ramsey of his day when he wrote *The Way to Wealth*. Within that text is this line: "There are no gains without pains."

Let me quote another favorite author. Paul, writer of the Book of Philippians, said, "I press toward the mark for the prize of the high calling of God in Christ Jesus" (Philippians 3:14).

And let me quote the author of *Porn in the Pew, 365 Days to Sexual Integrity, Porn-Free in 40 Days, A 90-Day Recovery Guide,* and *Jesus and the 12 Steps.* "To find lasting recovery, you must give up what you want *now* for that which you want *most*."

I find myself quoting myself with that one statement a lot. Why? Because it's true. As one country preacher said it, "That's where the rubber meets the wheel."

Acting out is always a choice in the moment. You can blame the "Big 3"—your trauma, abuse, and isolation. You can blame your mama, your papa, your environment, and the bully on the playground. But blame will get you nowhere. Get this through your head—*Every time you act out, it is a choice in the moment!*

You must answer this one question—every single time. *Is it worth it to sacrifice what I want most (a lifetime of recovery) for what I want now (a moment of pleasure)?*

Day 6
Only by Fasting

One day, a man brought his son to Jesus' disciples, hoping for a miracle. When they could not heal him, the boy was brought to Jesus. After Jesus drove a demon from the boy, the disciples asked why they had failed. Jesus said this kind of miracle was only possible after much "prayer and fasting" (Matthew 7:21).

What's the big deal about fasting? Matt Chandler provides an answer: "Fasting helps us reflect on the betterness of Jesus over all earthly pleasures."

Let me ask you a question. When was the last time you entered a period of fasting, while asking God to help you with your addiction? If you are married to a porn addict, have you fasted on his behalf, while seeking a miracle from God?

Fasting represents a level of commitment. Freedom is not the reward of the dabbler. If you dabble at therapy, 12-Step meetings, getting a sponsor, working the steps, or working an intense recovery program (such as my 90-day recovery program), you will come up short. If you are 90% committed, you are uncommitted.

Try it this week. Bring the two-barreled force of prayer and fasting into battle against your hurts, habits, and hang-ups.

Fasting represents sacrifice. It brings focus. It releases power. Fasting is the hidden weapon you have yet to employ. This might be a good time to start—if you really are serious about getting well. If you're not that serious, enjoy your next meal—while your struggles continue.

Day 7
Rise

St. Augustine said, "Do you want to rise? Begin by descending. Are you planning a tower that will pierce the clouds? Lay first the foundation of humility."

King David learned to rise in humility, but it didn't come quickly. As a young man, he prayed, "Don't let me suffer the fate of sinners; I am not like that" (Psalm 26:9).

As an older man, David prayed a different prayer. "I was born a sinner—yes, from the moment my mother conceived me" (Psalm 51:5).

Between those two prayers, David did some pretty cool things. But he didn't reach his full greatness until he admitted his full sinfulness. It's called humility, and it is a prerequisite to receiving the abundance of the blessings of God.

Let's end where we began, with a quote from Augustine. "It was pride that changed angels into devils; it is humility that makes men as angels."

If you have fallen to the depths of your addiction, take heart. You can rise. But you can't do it apart from humility.

Week 15
Mousetraps

"Mankind invented the bomb, but no mouse would ever construct a mousetrap."

- Albert Einstein

THIS WEEK'S EXERCISE
Find Your Cheese

Not all mice eat the same cheese. Actually, I'm not sure that's true, but it works for our purposes here. Ever since the days of Adam and Eve, we have all been enticed to indulge in things that bring instant gratification, but that threaten our spiritual lives. In the case of sexual temptations, this "cheese" will put our families and health at risk, as well.

In this exercise, you will deal with the cheese in your mousetrap by answering three questions.

Question #1—What "cheese" entices you the most? _____

_____

_____

Question #2—Why do you keep returning to the same trap? _____

_____

_____

_____

Question #3—How will you avoid this mousetrap in the future? _____

_____

_____

_____

Day 1
The Marshmallow Experiment

Perhaps you've heard of the Marshmallow Experiment. In the 1960s, a Stanford professor named Walter Mischel conducted an experiment with young children, ages four and five. They were each seated in a private room. Then Dr. Mischel placed a marshmallow on the table in front of them, with these directions. "I'm going to step out for a few minutes. I have placed a marshmallow in front of you. But if you can manage to not eat it until I get back, I'll give you a second marshmallow." Some took the marshmallow; others waited for the professor to return with a second marshmallow.

Years later, as these children matured, Dr. Mischel monitored their progress. He found that the children who waited for the second marshmallow scored higher on their SAT tests, had better social skills, and became more successful in life. In fact, 40 years later, they continued to live much more fulfilling lives.

Each day, you must answer one basic question: "Am I willing to pass on what I want *now* for what I want *most*?"

There was a man in the Bible named Esau. One day, he came home so hungry that he gave away his birthright to his younger brother in exchange for a bowl of soup. We are warned, "Make sure that no one is immoral or godless like Esau" (Hebrews 12:16).

Delayed gratification. It's not easy, but it's always better.

Inappropriate sexual activity is the marshmallow in the room. It can be yours pretty much anytime. But if you'll wait, God's blessings will be so much greater.

Day 2
When Nobody's Looking

J.C. Watt said, "Character is doing the right thing when nobody's looking."

If you are to find lasting recovery, you must learn to embrace activities that others will never see. It's called "doing the right things when nobody's looking."

In an article on sex addiction, Mara Tyler identifies four recovery activities many have found helpful: inpatient treatment programs, 12-Step groups, cognitive behavioral therapy, and medication. Those to whom you are closest—outside of immediate family—may never know you are doing any of these things. But if you are serious about recovery, you do them anyway.

Eventually, the things you are doing out of the sight of others will bring about the change that they will see. Paul said, "But all things become visible when they are exposed by the light, for everything that becomes visible is light" (Ephesians 5:13).

It's true that when you are in recovery, others will notice real change in your behavior. They will see you taking custody of your eyes, treating members of the opposite sex with respect, and avoiding compromising situations. But it is what you are doing that they cannot see that matters most.

Day 3
Thoughts

Gandhi said, "Your beliefs become your thoughts, your thoughts become your words, your words become your actions, your actions become your habits, your habits become your values, and your values become your destiny."

Norman Vincent Peale weighed in: "Change your thoughts and you change your world."

Finally, Paul wrote, "Be transformed by the renewing of your minds" (Romans 12:2).

Do you detect a theme that is a common thread in each of these quotes? Clearly, we do tomorrow what we think today. That is why it is so critical that we learn to manage our thoughts. Because your thoughts will dictate your behavior, you must learn to dictate your thoughts.

Take every thought captive. Make it a daily priority to restrict your thoughts to those things which are "true, noble, right, pure, lovely, and admirable" (Philippians 4:8).

The mind is one of the most deceiving mousetraps of all. There is no quicker way to get into trouble than with our thought lives. But you can find victory over your thoughts. Let me rephrase that. *You must find victory over your thoughts.*

Day 4
Porn Alert!

That God is all about sexual purity is pretty clear from Scripture. Paul wrote, "The body is not meant for sexual immorality, but for the Lord" (1 Corinthians

6:13). But pornography presents a beast of a mousetrap that is not easily overcome. Consider some recent studies.

Internet porn presents what sex researcher Dr. Alvin Cooper referred to as the "triple-A engine" of accessibility, affordability, and anonymity. The Web offers all three, which is a trap for the casual porn user.

How does this affect porn users? Drs. Destin Stewart and Dawn Szymanske, both of the University of Tennessee, conducted an extensive study on the effects of a man's porn use on his wife. They found that "those who perceived their husbands' (or boyfriends') porn use to be problematic experienced lower self-esteem, poorer relationship quality and lower sexual satisfaction."

Add a 2013 dual study by Brigham Young University and the University of Missouri. They surveyed heterosexual couples living together (married or not), where the men were frequent porn users. The result was "lower sexual quality for both the men and their partners."

The evidence is clear. God is against porn because porn is bad for us. The quicker we figure that out, the better off we'll be.

Take an honest look at the effects of porn on you and your relationships. Then respond accordingly.

Day 5
Get Creative

Albert Einstein said, "Creativity is intelligence having fun." Creativity may be the missing link to your recovery.

Doing the "intelligent" thing may not be enough. After all, it was your best thinking that got you into your mess in the first place. Perhaps it's time to step outside the boundaries of what has not been working. You might want to embrace the words of Pablo Picasso: "The chief enemy of creativity is good sense."

Seven hundred years before Christ, when his children were mired in predictability and apathy, God pronounced, "See, I am doing a new thing. I am making a way in the wilderness and streams in the wasteland" (Isaiah 43:18).

These "streams in the wasteland" went unseen until they were—*ready for some deep insight?*—seen. That required God's children to walk where they had never walked before.

To get where you have never been (recovery) you must walk where you have never gone.

Enter creativity.

I like the way Herman Melville said it. "It is better to fail in originality than to succeed in imitation." Application—God's plan for your recovery will not be exactly like anyone else's. To find your "streams in the wasteland," you must get creative. Seek a new path, a path that will require you to walk where you have never gone before.

Dieter Uchtdorf said, "The desire to create is one of the deepest yearnings of the human soul." Ask God for that desire. Seek the path of recovery that God has reserved just for you.

Day 6
Three Keys to Recovery

Every person who ever failed has the same thing in common. They quit too soon.

Tim Denning, author for Addicted2Success, writes, "Many people try something once and when they fail, they give up. That's because nobody tells you that achieving your dream doesn't happen the first time around."

This is especially true in recovery. I have yet to meet the man or woman who spent years acting out, suddenly walked into their first recovery meeting or therapy session, then walked out—never to act out again.

Solomon knew a little about success. He said, "A slack hand causes poverty, but the hand of the diligent makes rich" (Proverbs 10:4).

If you are struggling to maintain sobriety, I offer three suggestions:

1. Don't give up.
2. Don't give up.
3. Don't give up.

I have a friend with 25 years of sobriety. The key? "I didn't give up after the first ten years of failure," he says. Recovery is not a simple, point-by-point formula. It is part trial-and-error, part two steps forward and one step back, and mostly persistence. I promise you can get there—if you refuse to give up.

Day 7
A Single Punch

On November 5, 1994, Michael Moorer, the undefeated heavyweight champion of the world, stepped into the ring against 45-year-old George Foreman, who had not won a meaningful fight in nearly 20 years. Moorer led on all three judges' cards entering the final round. Then Foreman landed a single, devastating punch. Moorer went down. He would not get up.

Like Michael Moorer, in recovery, you can be ahead on points, and still go down with a single blow.

Complacency became the mousetrap that would do him in.

Jesus' close friend Peter serves as an astounding example of falling into that same trap.

"They took Jesus away, and Peter followed at a distance. When they had kindled a fire in the middle of the courtyard and sat down together, Peter sat down among them. Then a servant girl, seeing him as he sat in the light and looking closely at him, said, 'This man also was with him.' But Peter denied it, saying, 'Woman, I do not know him'" (Luke 22:54-57).

No matter how close you are to Jesus, a single sin can bring you down. That is why the great baseball player turned preacher Billy Sunday said, "I'm against sin. I'll kick it as long as I've got a foot, and I'll fight it as long as I've got a fist. I'll butt it as long as I've got a head, and I'll bite it as long as I've got a tooth. And when I'm old and fistless and footless and toothless, I'll gum it till I go home to glory and it goes home to perdition!"

May each of us resist the temptations of sin with the same conviction!

Week 16
Forgiveness

*"Always forgive your enemies. Nothing
will annoy them more."*

- Ocsar Wilde

THIS WEEK'S EXERCISE
Write a Letter to Yourself

In recovery, it is imperative that we learn to forgive those who have injured us with the "big 3"—abuse, trauma, and isolation. But there is another person we need to forgive. That is, of course, ourselves. For many, this seems a bridge too far. When we look back at all we have done to hurt our spouse, children, and those closest to us, we can retreat into the sea of shame, never to be heard from again.

If you have struggled with sexually compulsive activity, this is not an option. You must forgive yourself.

This is a form of making amends. And as with other amends, it is best done in writing. So your exercise this week is to write a letter to yourself. God has already forgiven you, so now it's your turn. Forgive yourself for all that you have done and all whom you have hurt. And pledge to walk a different path for the rest of your life—one day at a time.

Write your letter here.

_____

_____

_____

_____

_____

_____

_____

_____

_____

_____

_____

Day 1
Resentment

Recovery is incomplete until we deal with our resentments.

In *Wishful Thinking*, Pastor Frederick Buechner wrote about the effects of bitterness on a man harboring resentment. "Of the seven deadly sins, anger is the most fun. To lick your wounds, to smack your lips over grievances long past, to savor to the last morsel both the pain you are given and the pain you are giving back—in many ways it is a feast fit for a king. The only drawback is that what you are wolfing down is yourself. The skeleton at the feast is you!"

Jesus was clear. "Whenever you stand praying, forgive, if you have anything against anyone, so that your Father also who is in heaven may forgive you your trespasses" (Mark 11:25).

Against whom do you harbor resentments? Your parents? A pastor? Your spouse? Maybe even God? Regardless of how justified you think you are in your resentments, you must let them go. They are only killing you. And they make a full recovery impossible.

The good news is, forgiveness is actually easier than resentment. M.L. Stedman explains. In her 2012 novel, *The Light Between Oceans*, Stedman writes, "You only have to forgive once. To resent, you have to do it all day, every day."

It's up to you. You can forgive once or resent all day, every day—whichever you think makes the most sense.

Day 2
Houdini

Harry Houdini decided to take his show to a whole new level. He had escaped jail cells, straitjackets under water, and an oversized milk can filled with water. He had accomplished his latest stunt numerous times—jumping off bridges into the water below while handcuffed. But on August 26, 1907, he plunged into the water—bound by chains. As a mortified audience looked on, it took him 57 seconds to break free.

The Bible tells us about a man named Legion, who had "often been chained" (Mark 5:4). He would cut himself with stones while running through cemeteries. Some found him scary. Others thought he was possessed by demons. The clinical diagnosis is obvious. The dude was nuts.

Enter one Messiah into the picture. "When he saw Jesus from a distance, he ran and fell on his knees in front of him" (5:6). That changed everything.

Germany Kent said, "Don't live the same day over and over again and call that a life."

Are you ready to quit living the same day over and over again? Are you ready to break free of the chains that bind you?

If you're ready for real change, do what the man in the cemetery did. Come to Jesus, and forgive yourself for all the crazy things in your past.

Day 3
The Golden Rule

In his book of semi-philosophical and satirical stories titled *Fuzzy Memories*, Jack Handey writes, "There used to be this bully who would demand my lunch money every day. Since I was smaller, I would give it to him. But then I decided to fight back. I started taking karate lessons. Then the karate lesson guy said I had to start paying him five dollars a lesson. So I just went back to paying the bully."

Most addicts were bullied on some level as children. It may have been physical abuse or a form of emotional abuse that went undetected. As adults, we become that bully. It's all we know. We do unto others as has been done unto us.

Jesus prescribed a better medicine. "In everything, do to others what you would have them do to you, for this sums up the Law and the Prophets" (Matthew 7:12).

Tony Campolo is right when he suggests, "Each of us comes into the world with a predisposition to live in such a way as to inflict pain on those who love us most, and to offend the God who cares for us infinitely."

Our recovery is largely dependent upon how we treat others. When the bullied becomes the bully, the unhealthy cycle continues. But it can stop with you. Now.

Day 4
The Wounded Spouse

If you are the wounded spouse, one of the toughest mountains you will ever climb will be Mt. Forgiveness. In forgiving your mate, you relinquish all rights to retribution and payback. You accept him or her as though they had never abandoned you for the selfishness of their addiction.

Forgiveness may not seem fair. But it is necessary. Absolutely necessary—for your own healing.

Ephesians 4:31 says, "Get rid of all bitterness, rage and anger, brawling and slander, along with every form of malice."

In other words, forgive the one who has hurt you the most. Bryant McGill was right when he said, "There is no love without forgiveness, and there is no forgiveness without love."

Legendary wrestler Lex Lugar has a lot of regrets. But he has found hope in Christ. A few years ago, he reflected on his life. "Many times, the decisions we make affect and hurt our closest friends and family the most. I have a lot of regrets in that regard. But God has forgiven me, which I am very grateful for. It has enabled me to forgive myself and move forward one day at a time."

Has your spouse wounded you? You need to forgive him or her. Don't do it for them. Do it for you.

Day 5
The One You Need to Forgive the Most

In the movie *Spider-Man 3*, Peter Parker spoke this famous line: "You want forgiveness? Get religion."

The fact is, we all want forgiveness. The sad thing is that we are more prone to offer our forgiveness to others than we are to forgive ourselves. The answer? Stay at it.

Paul said, "We glory in our sufferings, because we know that suffering produces perseverance" (Romans 5:3).

Forgiveness of self is the picture of perseverance. We grow impatient with ourselves as we continue to commit the same sins over and over. We relapse. We slip. We vow, "Never again!" And then it happens. Again and again—it happens.

Jesus said to forgive 490 times (Matthew 18:22). I suggest that if this is to be our mindset toward others, it should be our mindset toward ourselves, first. After all, we are told to love others *as we love ourselves* (Matthew 22:39).

Slips do not need to result in shame. A relapse is not the end, but a beginning. And that beginning starts by forgiving yourself, just as God already has.

Day 6
Vengeance

Two little brothers, Harry and Jimmy, had finished supper and were playing until bedtime. Somehow, Harry hit Jimmy with a stick, and tears and bitter words followed. Charges and accusations were still being exchanged as Mother prepared them for bed. She said, "Now, Jimmy, before you go to bed you're going to have to forgive your brother."

Jimmy was thoughtful, and then replied, "Well, okay, I'll forgive him tonight, but if I don't die before I wake up, he'd better look out in the morning."

It is natural to seek revenge on those who have hurt us—but it is never healthy.

Rodney King said, "I'm a religious person. I remember my mom told me, 'Vengeance belongs to God. It's up to him to wreak vengeance.' It's hard for me to get to that point, but that's the work of God."

You are the product of the harms done to you by others. You can't help what has been done to you. But you are responsible for how you respond.

1 Peter 3:9 says, "Do not repay evil with evil or insult with insult. On the contrary, repay evil with blessings, because to this you were called so that you may inherit a blessing."

Day 7
Time to Move On

Philadelphia Phillies centerfielder Richie Ashburn could foul pitches off at will, but one day he got a little carried away. During a game against the New York Giants in 1957, Ashburn slapped a foul ball that struck a fan in the stands. The ball hit Alice Roth squarely in the face, breaking her nose. Then things got even worse. As medics carried her away on a stretcher, Ashburn hit another foul ball into the stands—this time striking Roth a second time, in the leg.

Roth's husband was Earl Roth, the sports editor for the *Philadelphia Bulletin*. When Ashburn became eligible for the baseball Hall of Fame, Roth remembered those foul balls, and he voted against Ashburn 15 years in a row.

At the genesis of most addictions is trauma. For the sex addict, that means someone brought him or her some level of abuse: physical, emotional, or sexual. In recovery, one of the biggest steps one must take is that of forgiveness. Every person who realizes successful recovery has learned to forgive those who hurt them the most.

Paul identified the weapon missing from most of our arsenals—forgiveness. His words are unambiguous: "Forgive each other as the Lord has forgiven you" (Colossians 3:13).

If you have struggled with porn or sex addiction, there probably is someone in your past who harmed you deeply. You have traveled the road of resentment long enough. It's time to take the exit ramp of forgiveness.

Week 17
Temptation

"I generally avoid temptation unless I can resist it."

- Mae West

THIS WEEK'S EXERCISE
Beat Back Temptation

When temptation comes knocking on your door, you need a plan. You can answer the door and let it in. Or you can keep the door locked. What you cannot do is hide in the back room, pretending you aren't at home. You must respond.

But if you wait until the knock on the door before you have a plan in place, you will be playing with fire. You need a three-phase plan for dealing with temptation: (a) what to do **before** the temptation hits, (b) what to do **when** the temptation hits, and (c) what to do **after** the temptation hits.

Before the Temptation Hits

You know it's coming. There is no chance that you will be immune to temptation. The enemy is real, and he wants to bring you down. Your own past makes you vulnerable to certain attacks. But the good news is that you can prepare for the enemy. You would be foolish to not prepare. So what are some of the steps you will take in advance, to put yourself in the best possible position for victory, when the temptation hits?

- _____
- _____
- _____
- _____
- _____

When the Temptation Hits

While there are certainly steps you can take to avoid temptation and to prepare for temptation, there will be times when temptation will be unavoidable. You need to be ready for these moments. You can do everything right, and still get hit out of the blue with an intrusive thought, physical temptation, or trigger. What are some steps you will take to respond when temptation hits?

- _____
- _____
- _____
- _____
- _____

After the Temptation Hits

At some point this week, you will face temptation. You need to learn from that temptation, whether you gave into it or not. So think about your most recent sexual temptation, and reflect on some lessons you can take away from that situation.

- _____
- _____
- _____
- _____
- _____

Day 1
Why God Allows Temptation

J.I. Packer wrote the classic book, *Knowing God*. On the subject of personal hardships in the Christian's life, Packer states, "God exposes us to these things, so as to overwhelm us with a sense of our own inadequacy, and to drive us to cling to him more closely. This is the ultimate reason, from our standpoint, why God fills our lives with troubles and perplexities of one sort or another—it is to ensure that we shall learn to hold him fast."

One of those perplexities is the temptations that keep coming, despite endless moments of remorse, repentance, and recommitments.

You are promised, "No temptation has overtaken you except what is common to mankind. And God is faithful; he will not let you be tempted beyond what you can bear. But when you are tempted, he will also provide a way out so that you can endure it" (1 Corinthians 10:13).

When you face temptation, you have two choices. You can (a) give in, or (b) look up. In our addictions, we need to learn to look up. We must see temptation as a test. Each time we pass the test, we gain new strength for the next time.

Today, when you are tempted, follow Packer's advice. Let that temptation "drive you to cling to him more closely . . . learn to hold him fast."

Day 2
Sex and Ice Cream

I still remember my first "fix." I was in my late 20s. I'm not sure how I discovered my new "drug," but when I did, I was hooked. From the first time I indulged, the image has been firmly lodged in my mind—for more than 30 years. Sometimes, I have gone several months without my "drug," while other times, I only abstain for a few days at a time. But the image is always there.

I'm talking, of course, about a strawberry soda from LaKing's Ice Cream Parlor in Galveston, Texas. They do it the old-fashioned way. To step into LaKing's is to step into 1920s America. They make their own taffy, candy, and strawberry sodas. I've been known to down three of them in one setting. And then I'm satisfied—for a day or two. No matter how many strawberry sodas I've had, I always want one more.

I identify with Oscar Wilde, who said, "I can resist anything except temptation."

Whether it is ice cream, tobacco, alcohol, or sex, we become slaves to our appetites. And then they own us. But it doesn't have to be that way.

Paul determined, "I will not be mastered by anything" (1 Corinthians 6:12).

The temptations do not go away. The key is to see that as an opportunity, and not a trap. As Ralph Waldo Emerson wrote, "We gain strength through the temptations we resist." Sometimes, it's as simple as that. We must learn to resist, to not give in. Each day we do that, we get just a little bit stronger.

Day 3
After the Temptation

Overcoming temptation is the focus of any person's sobriety. But what comes after the temptation must not be ignored.

The Bible tells us that "Jesus was led by the Spirit into the wilderness to be tempted by the devil. After fasting forty days and forty nights, he was hungry" (Matthew 4:1-2).

I see two lessons here.

First, we can be at risk *after* the temptation, not just *before* it. Jesus became hungry. Hunger takes us to a place of vulnerability.

Second, while the temptation can be exhausting, victory gives us strength and confidence for the next battle. John Bunyan said it like this: "Temptations, when we meet them at first, are as the lion that roared upon Samson, but if we overcome them, the next time we see them we shall find a nest of honey within them."

Temptation is a battle we all must face. But don't lose focus—because what comes next matters just as much.

Day 4
Before You Relapse

All over the world, every hour of every day, addicts of all kinds do it. They relapse. For many addicts, there is a never-ending search for a silver bullet—that one trick that will keep the addict sober in the heat of the moment.

There are no silver bullets. Sorry to inform you of that. But there are a few things you can and should do before you slip or relapse. The next time you feel a strong compulsion to act out, consult this list. Do these things . . . before you relapse.

1. Pray the Serenity Prayer.
2. Pray the Third Step Prayer.
3. Make a call.
4. Play your pending action forward in your head—how does it end?
5. Read recovery material.
6. Read some Scripture.
7. Make a gratitude list.
8. Work one of the 12 steps.

Then try this—my personal gem. Practice the 20-minute rule. Hold out for 20 minutes, and you can purge the urge. The height of temptation will pass in 20 minutes. If you can stay sober for just 20 minutes—and you can—then you can stay sober for the rest of the day.

The Bible promises us that we can escape every temptation. To not do so is a choice. The next time you feel tempted to act out, consider the list above . . . before you relapse.

Day 5
Duplicity

In the semifinals of the 1982 French Open, Mats Wilander was the overwhelming favorite, playing on clay, which was his favorite surface. It was match point, when his opponent hit a ball down the line. The ball was ruled out, and Wilander advanced to the finals.

But not so quick. Wilander approached the chair umpire and said, "I can't win like this. The ball was good." The point was played over, and Wilander won fair and square.

The Bible says, "The integrity of the upright guides them, but the unfaithful are destroyed by their duplicity" (Proverbs 11:3).

Integrity is a good motivation for recovery. When I got into serious recovery, something else happened. I started looking better in the mirror. I could look at myself with pride, knowing I was no longer living the life which Solomon calls "duplicity."

Are you tired of living the life of duplicity—one life in private and another in public? Then go all in with recovery.

President Dwight Eisenhower said it well: "The supreme quality for leadership is unquestionably integrity." And you can't live a life of integrity and duplicity at the same time.

Day 6
Johnny Mercer

One day in 1956, songwriter Johnny Mercer received a letter from Sadie Vimmerstedt, a widowed grandmother who worked behind a cosmetics counter in Youngstown, Ohio. Vimmerstedt suggested that Mercer write a song called *I Want to Be Around to Pick Up the Pieces When Somebody Breaks Your Heart*.

Five years later, Mercer wrote the song and Tony Bennett agreed to record it. Today, if you look at the label on any recording of *I Wanna Be Around*, you will notice the credits for the words are shared by Mercer and Vimmerstedt. The royalties were split 50-50, due to the generous honesty of Johnny Mercer.

By offering Mrs. Vimmerstedt half of the royalties, her family has made $100,000 and counting.

Johnny Mercer practiced what Jesus called "doing for others what you would want them to do for you" (Matthew 7:12).

Let's put a different twist on this story. Are you so committed to your personal integrity that you will do the right things, whether anyone else sees that or not? Or to make it more personal, would you ever look at porn again, if there were no consequences?

Well, guess what? There are consequences—always. The problem with secret choices is not what they do to us, but what they create in us.

It's what you do that you don't have to do that counts. Living in freedom and integrity means doing the right thing—when no one is watching.

Day 7
Finish the Task

A lot of people begin the work of recovery, but fail to complete it. There is a book in the Bible written on this subject. That book is Zechariah. Here's the story.

God's people had returned to Israel, on the heels of their captivity in Babylon. Following the leadership of Ezra and Nehemiah, they had begun to rebuild their lives as well as their Temple. But they failed to complete the task. So God sent them two prophets—Haggai and Zechariah—to challenge them to step up to the challenge.

God's command to finish the work was accompanied with a promise: "I promise this very day that I will repay two blessings for each of your troubles" (Zechariah 9:12).

The theme of Zechariah is heart change. God repeatedly warned his children that he did not put much value in their fasts, feasts, and outward signs of devotion. It was the attitude of the heart that mattered most.

The same is true for us. While it is important to engage in specific recovery activities—attending meetings, getting a sponsor, working the 12 Steps, going to therapy—it is the condition of your heart that concerns your God.

And that is where the battle with temptation is won—in the heart.

Week 18
Community

"God has called me into a personal relationship with his Son,
but he hasn't called me into a private relationship with his Son."

- Anonymous

THIS WEEK'S EXERCISE
Name a Pair

Dr. Dennis Swanberg has given us some great insight into the value of community in *The Man Code*. He delves into the example of Jesus and the groups that mattered to him on a personal level. Among those, Jesus had a group of three (his inner circle), a group of 12 (his small group), and a group of 120 (which represents the church).

Likewise, we need certain people in our sphere of influence and fellowship. You were not created to be alone, and you cannot sustain recovery by yourself. When you talk to guys who have been in 12-Step groups for years, you will hear a myriad of reasons guys are in the program: (a) 12-Step work, (b) working with a sponsor, (c) reading through the materials. But the thing you will hear most is that the men draw great strength and encouragement from being with other guys who share the same struggle.

We all need community. But not all community is good. Today, focus on the people you need to embrace in your life, as well as those you need to avoid.

Avoid? Yes! We all know people who are simply too toxic to be in our inner circle, or even in our lives at all. They bring us down. They may be bad triggers or a negative influence. As important as it is to fellowship with the right people, we need to walk away from the wrong people. They aren't necessarily bad people, but they are bad for us.

Exercise #1—The Right Crowd

List up to five people you need to seek time with, who will help move your recovery forward.

- _____
- _____
- _____
- _____
- _____

Exercise #2—The Wrong Crowd

List up to five people who are toxic, and who you need to not have in your life right now.

- _____
- _____
- _____
- _____
- _____

Day 1
It Takes a Team

Congratulations on your commitment to personal purity! There are two truths you must embrace early on: community and transparency.

Dietrich Bonhoeffer wrote, in *Life Together*, "The final obstacle to true Christian fellowship is the inability to be sinners together."

We must learn to be together, but togetherness is not enough. Sobriety is dependent on connecting with saints who know they are sinners. Then we must become comfortable with being sinners together.

It is impossible to overstate the need for transparent community in recovery. Alex Lerza, clinical psychologist and Certified Sex Addiction Therapist, says it like this: "The opposite of addiction is not sobriety, but relationship."

The secret sauce for the early church was their interconnectedness. "They devoted themselves to the apostles' teaching and the fellowship" (Acts 2:42). Most churches are big on teaching but weak on fellowship. We need both.

Find a group with whom you can connect at the deepest levels of life. How will you know you have found the right group? They are comfortable with being sinners together.

Day 2
That's What Friends Are For

In 1985, Dionne Warwick recorded one of her most popular songs, *That's What Friends Are For*. The closing lines are:

"Keep smiling, keep shining
Knowing you can always count on me, for sure
Cause I tell you, that's what friends are for
Whoa, good times and the bad times
I'll be on your side forever more
That's what friends are for."

Your real friends stick with you, not because you are good but because you are bad. Pick your friends carefully. Why? Because after you make friends, they will make you.

The Bible warns, "Walk with the wise and become wise; associate with fools and get in trouble" (Proverbs 13:20).

Surround yourself, in recovery and in life, with people who will love you on your worst day. For each of us, there are times when we cannot take the next step on our own. And that's okay, because . . .

That's what friends are for.

Ask God to bring two or three people into your life with whom you can share your deepest valleys and darkest moments. After all, *that's what friends are for.*

Day 3
Established

D.L. Moody, famed 19th century evangelist, told the story of a man who was asked by his young son why he didn't go to church. His dad explained, "I don't need to go to church, son. My faith is established." Later that day, the man drove his horses out of the barn and hitched them to the buggy. As they drove them out of the yard, the horses became mired in a mud hole. The boy said, "Daddy, I don't think the horses are going anywhere. They are established."

"Established" is just another word for "stuck." And that's what happens to our spiritual development when we abandon the fellowship of the local church—we get stuck.

The Bible warns us, "Don't neglect your fellowship together, as has become the habit of some" (Hebrews 10:25).

Recovery is all about breaking old habits and learning new ones. Dr. Susan McQuillan, noted psychologist, says, "We keep doing the wrong thing because it is impossible to unlearn a bad habit on our own."

Recovery never happens in isolation. In fact, it is isolation that gets us in trouble in the first place. You need others along the journey. And you need to be in church. Otherwise, your recovery will stall out. You will become stuck.

Day 4
Don't Stand Alone

He was the world's most famous recluse, the hermit's hermit, and the richest man alive. His name was Howard Hughes. An aviator, industrialist, and film producer, Hughes began showing signs of mental illness while in his 30s. On Thanksgiving Day of 1966, he moved into a suite at Las Vegas' Desert Inn. He refused to leave his room. When they insisted he leave, he bought the hotel. Howard Hughes never found the peace that comes from healthy relationships. Fittingly, ten years later, he died alone.

We were never intended to do life alone. Few find recovery on their own. Gandhi said, "The best way to find yourself is to lose yourself in service to others." The man who stands alone will surely fall.

An elderly lady stood in line at the post office once a week, to buy stamps. The line often took about 30 minutes. An employee noted this pattern and approached the lady one day. "You do know you can buy your stamps from the stamp machine, don't you? Why do you stand in line for 30 minutes when you could get them so much quicker?"

The lady replied, "It's simple. When I get to the counter, the young man working there speaks to me. But that stupid stamp machine never says a word."

We need others in order to win the race of life. That's why Solomon wrote, "Though one may be overpowered, two can defend themselves. A cord of three strands is not quickly broken" (Ecclesiastes 4:12).

Day 5
Friends

It premiered on September 22, 1994. After a ten-year run on NBC, after 236 episodes, the show concluded its run on May 6, 2004, before an audience of 52.5 million. Of course, I'm talking about *Friends*, a series centered around the relationships of six friends. Winner of 62 Primetime Emmys, the show is ranked #21 on TV Guide's list of the top 50 television shows of all-time.

Everybody needs a friend. A recent Gallup Poll found that the average person has nine friends. Sadly, about 10 percent have none. And that's a problem, according to Patrick Allan, author of *This Is How Many Friends You Need to Be Happy*. Allan writes, "Isolation and loneliness are the killers of today's generation."

If you are an addict, or married to one, you need friends. They don't necessarily need to be endowed with great wisdom. They just need to care. Henri Nouwen said, "The friend who can be silent with us in a moment of despair or confusion, who can stay with us in an hour of grief and bereavement, who can tolerate not knowing, not healing, not curing, that is a friend who cares."

The Book of 2 Kings describes just such a friend. His name was Elisha. When Naaman, a Syrian general, looked him up, Elisha became the friend he didn't ask for, but desperately needed. Naaman had been stricken with leprosy. Elisha told him exactly what to do: "Go wash seven times in the Jordan and your skin will be restored and you will be clean" (5:10).

Sometimes a friend—like Elisha—says things that don't make much sense. But in the most desperate cases—as with Naaman—it works out. I know two things about you. You need to find a friend like that, and you need to be a friend like that.

Day 6
Community

According to Dr. Adrian Hickmon, founder of Capstone, there are two essentials to early recovery work: a therapist and a community. Let's talk about the second component—community.

Paul wrote, "Carry each other's burdens, and in this way you will fulfill the law of Christ" (Galatians 6:2).

There is a popular saying in AA: "I can't stay sober, but we can."

Empirical data confirms the need for community.

Kathlene Tracy and Samantha Wallace consulted ten studies on successful recovery models over the past 20 years. They concluded that each one had as a primary component "peer support groups." Their findings can be found in the Community Research and Recovery Program in the Department of Psychiatry at the New York University School of Medicine.

Here's the simple conclusion—you can find recovery, but you can't find it on your own.

Identify an individual and a group (such as Sexaholics Anonymous or Celebrate Recovery) which you will intentionally include in your personal recovery plan.

Day 7
Four Core Beliefs

There are four core beliefs of every addict: (a) Something is wrong with me. (b) If you knew me, you wouldn't love me. (c) I am alone. (d) My addictive behavior is my greatest need.

Let's talk about that second one—if you knew me, you wouldn't love me. That's a real bummer, because we all long to be loved.

Oprah Winfrey said, "Lots of people want to ride with you in the limo, but what you want is someone who will take the bus with you when the limo breaks down."

Walter Winchell said it like this: "A real friend is one who walks in when the rest of the world walks out."

Recovery is a team sport. You can't get there on your own. You need others in your life who will love you as much on your worst day as on your best, whether you fall or rise, when you slip and when you get up.

The Scripture is emphatic. "A friend loves at *all* times" (Proverbs 17:17). All means all.

If you are new to recovery, find a friend like that. If you are further along in your recovery, be a friend like that.

Week 19
Markers

"Our goals should serve as markers, measurements of the progress we make in pursuit of something greater than ourselves."

- Simon Sinek

THIS WEEK'S EXERCISE
What Phase Are You In?

It is important that you understand where you are in your recovery process and where you are headed. Some experts, such as Patrick Carnes and Milton Magness, have taught that the full process of recovery is measured in years, usually about three to five.

Milton Magness lists four phases of recovery.

Phase 1—Survival (six months to one year)

You are in the Survival Phase of your recovery if you:
- Have just started your recovery
- Have recently slipped or relapsed
- Have not been able to establish a period of sobriety
- Have recently experienced a crisis related to acting out

Phase 2—Stability (six months to two years)

This is a period when you begin to find sure footing in your recovery. You are in the Stability Phase of your recovery if you:

- Have established sobriety
- Have good recovery routines established including attending 12-Step meetings
- Are actively working with a sponsor

Phase 3—Sustaining (18 months to three years)

This phase usually begins between 18 months and three years into recovery and lasts one year or more. You are in this phase if you:

- Have made a disclosure of your acting out behaviors to your relationship partner
- Are successfully living "slip free," with unbroken sobriety of at least six months
- Your partner is actively working his or her own recovery

Phase 4—Freedom (2.5 years or more)

This is the maintenance phase of recovery, and this is momentous! This comes after 2.5 years or more of recovery work. Here, you are moving away from regular therapy and finding victory. You are in this stage if you:

- Have at least one year of unbroken sobriety
- Are living a balanced, growing life
- Have reached the point in which acting out has become more of a memory than a present temptation

Here's your exercise. First, identify which phase you are in today. Second, explain how you plan to move forward into the next phase.

Your current phase of recovery

- Survival Phase _____
- Stability Phase _____
- Sustaining Phase _____
- Freedom Phase _____

Now, explain how you plan to move to the next phase. (If you are in the Freedom Phase, explain how you plan to stay there.)

_____

_____

_____

_____

_____

_____

_____

Day 1
Celebrate Success!

Early in recovery, it is natural for an addict to look around the room in a 12-Step meeting and conclude, "There are guys here with years of sobriety! I have so far to go!"

We need to celebrate early success in our recovery. In the Old Testament we read about the determination that led the Israelites to rebuild the Temple, their sacred place of worship. "When the builders completed the foundation of the Lord's Temple, they clashed their cymbals to praise the Lord, just as King David had prescribed" (Ezra 3:10).

Did you catch that? The builders didn't hold off the celebration until the Temple was finished. They celebrated when the Temple was *started*.

Recovery is never finished. If you wait until you have reached perfection, until you have "arrived" to celebrate, you can leave the cymbals in the box.

The fact that you are reading this right now is something. Even the smallest of steps in early recovery are to be celebrated. If you attend a 12-Step meeting, you will hear about the 24-hour desire chip. When someone claims that chip, they are committing to sobriety for the next 24 hours—not 24 days, weeks, or years.

The builders celebrated the laying of the foundation of the Temple. You have begun to lay a foundation on which to build a life of recovery. That's huge! Take time to celebrate!

Day 2
12 Stones

God's children had dreamed of reaching the Promised Land for generations. Finally, under the leadership of Joshua, that day came. And they were quick to commemorate the event. Joshua told the men to set stones in place as a memorial of the crossing of the Jordan River. And then he told them what to tell the next generation.

"Tell them that the flow of the Jordan was cut off before the ark of the covenant of the Lord. When it crossed the Jordan, the waters of the Jordan were cut off. These stones are to be a memorial to the people of Israel forever" (Joshua 4:7).

The children of God still had a long way to go, but this was a day to remember how far they had already come. They didn't have much, but they were headed in the right direction.

In recovery, it is important to remember what we have already achieved, with the help of God.

Charles Spurgeon said, "It is not how much we have, but how much we enjoy that makes us happy."

Sure, you still have a long way to go. But today, be thankful for how far you have already come.

Day 3
Dance to the Music

In 1975 Three Dog Night released one of their biggest hits. The lyrics follow.

"Slippin' away, sittin' on a pillow
Waitin' for night to fall.
A girl and a dream, sittin' on a pillow
This is the night to go to the celebrity ball.

Celebrate, celebrate, dance to the music.
Celebrate, celebrate, dance to the music.
Celebrate, celebrate, dance to the music."

It had been a long, 40-year journey through the wilderness. God's children had finally figured it out and reached the Promised Land. First, there was a river to cross. Once on the other side, it was time to celebrate. Their leader spoke up.

"Each of you is to take up a stone on his shoulder, according to the number of tribes of the Israelites. These stones are to be a memorial to the people of Israel forever" (Joshua 4:5, 7).

By carefully placing the stones, they paused to celebrate how far they had come before taking another step. If you have had even one day of sobriety, you have something to celebrate. So go ahead. Dance to the music.

Day 4
Wrong Definition

Dr. Adrian Hickmon says, "Measuring how spiritual a person is by the level of their addiction is like measuring a person's height with a bathroom scale."

Always take your addiction seriously, but never let it define you. A common statement in recovery goes like this: "I am not defined by my relapses, but by my decision to remain in recovery despite them."

Perhaps you have experienced numerous slips and relapses since you started down the path to recovery. That is not uncommon. But as Winston Churchill famously said, "Never, ever, ever, ever, ever give up."

There was a man in the New Testament named John Mark. He joined Paul on his first missionary journey. But he quickly flamed out. A few years later, Mark was ready to jump back in, but Paul wouldn't give him a chance. Why? Because Paul defined him by his failure.

But one man believed in Mark—cousin Barnabas. Because Barnabas believed in Mark, Mark could believe in himself. The result was threefold: (a) Mark would have a productive career as a missionary, (b) Paul would come to recognize him as a "fellow worker" (Colossians 4:10), and (c) Mark would write the Gospel of Mark.

Not a bad life for a failure.

Day 5
Comeback Stories

I love a good comeback story: the 1951 Giants coming from 13 games back to win the pennant, the 1993 Bills coming from 35 points down to beat the Oilers, 45-year old George Foreman coming back to win the heavyweight championship of the world.

Every successful person has a comeback story. In fact, the Bible is full of them: Noah, Moses, David, Paul, and Peter.

If you have fallen, you can become a comeback story. God stands perfectly positioned to turn your set-back into his set-up.

But he won't do it without your participation. J. Paul Getty said it well. "My formula for success is to rise early, work late, and strike oil."

Paul said, "Forgetting my past, I strive for what is ahead" (Philippians 3:13).

I don't know your story, but I do know your God. And I know this—nothing in your past is bad enough or strong enough to stop God from leading you into an amazing future.

Day 6
Not Enough

Jim Carrey was right: "I think everybody should get rich and famous and do everything they ever dreamed of so they can see it's not the answer."

That's a pretty powerful statement considering the source. If anyone had enough riches and fame to be happy, it would be Jim Carrey. His resume is pretty impressive:

- Net worth of $150 million
- Two Golden Globe Awards
- One Grammy nomination
- Four People's Choice Awards

Still, the iconic movie star suffers from depression. He knows what it is to have ridiculous wealth and fame. And he knows they are not "the answer."

The world's wealthiest man agreed. Solomon said, "He who trusts in his riches will fall, but the righteous will flourish like the green leaf" (Proverbs 11:28).

What are you trusting in? Jim Carrey can tell you money and popularity aren't the answer. And I can tell you the answer is not sex. I have discovered what Solomon discovered. The answer is in God. St. Augustine said it so well: "Thou hast made us for thyself, O Lord, and our heart is restless until it finds rest in thee."

Day 7
When It's a Good Idea to Look Back

Will Rogers said, "Don't let yesterday use up too much of today."

The prophet warned, "Remember not the former things, nor consider the things of old" (Isaiah 43:18).

These statements underscore a sound principle. I like to use the car illustration. We have a large windshield so we can look forward for most of the drive, but a small rearview mirror, so we can glance back from time to time.

But never underestimate the value of glancing back.

Several years ago, my sponsor gave me some great advice. He said recovery is like climbing a mountain. We need to look forward in order to climb higher. But we should also glance down from time to time to see how far we've come.

Take a glance back. See how far you've come. Sure, you still have a long way to go. We all do. But don't let your view into the journey ahead take away from the ground you have already conquered.

Keep your eye on the prize. But you should also take time to celebrate the victories you have already won.

Week 20
Middle Circle

"Middle circle behaviors tend to lead addicts

back to the inner circle."

\- Sex Addicts Anonymous

THIS WEEK'S EXERCISE
Update Your Middle Circle

Of the three circles (outer, middle, inner), this is the most important and the one that changes the most. While the outer circle represents those behaviors that contribute to your sobriety and the inner circle behaviors are those which represent a breach in your sobriety, it is the middle circle that determines your destiny. These are the things you do that, while not breaking your sobriety, lead you dangerously close to the inner circle behaviors that represent relapse.

It is wisest to enlist the help of a sponsor or someone else with strong sobriety, before completing your middle circle list. And again, this will be fluid. There will be some activities you can move out of the middle circle eventually, and other activities you will need to add.

Here are a few examples of common middle circle activities:

- Watching certain TV channels or shows
- Staying up too late at night
- Too much time on social media
- Browsing the Internet
- Dropping out of 12-Step meetings
- An unhealthy diet
- Toxic relationships
- Time that is not accounted for
- Traveling alone
- Lunch with someone of the opposite sex
- Certain music
- Unprotected devices
- Texting with the opposite sex
- Carrying too much cash
- Particular restaurants, malls, or areas of town

List your middle circle behaviors:

- _____
- _____
- _____
- _____
- _____
- _____

Day 1
Progressive Porn

Mark Wayne Salling was a successful actor and musician. He was admired for his role as Noah "Puck" Puckerman on the television series Glee. But on December 29, 2015, Salling was arrested at his Los Angeles home on suspicion of possessing thousands of photos and videos of child pornography. Over 50,000 photos were eventually found. Salling was officially charged on May 27, 2016. On September 30, 2017, he pled guilty and was registered as a sex offender. He faced four to seven years in prison, and his sentencing date was set for March 2018. But three months before his sentencing date, on December 18, 2017, Mark Salling hung himself near his home.

Porn will take you further than you want to go, keep you longer than you want to stay, and cost you more than you want to pay.

Paul said it in simple terms: "The wages of sin is death" (Romans 6:23).

One of the scary truths about addiction is that it is progressive. Rarely does a man dabble in porn, then stop on his own—without intervention. That intervention may take the form of an arrest, a broken marriage, or some other price to pay.

What we dabble in becomes our "middle circle" behaviors. As first described by Alcoholics Anonymous, these are the things in which we indulge which lead us down a path of destruction.

If you are "dabbling" in porn, read the first paragraph again. Let the tragedy of Mark Wayne Salling's life be a warning to you.

Day 2
Mired in the Weeds

The date was October 13, 1960. Andy Jerke was just like every other boy growing up in Pittsburgh. He loved baseball, and especially the Pirates. On this day, the Pirates were hosting the vaunted New York Yankees for Game 7 of the World Series. The game came down to the bottom of the ninth inning. The score was tied. And Andy was there, at Forbes Field.

Then he remembered he had promised his mother to be home by 4:30 to help with dinner. So he left the game in the bottom of the ninth, to walk home.

As he was walking across the lot beyond the outfield wall, a baseball landed near his feet. Andy picked up the ball, and a security man informed him that Bill

Mazeroski had just hit that ball for a game-winning home run. And now the ball belonged to Andy.

Andy played with the ball a year later and lost it in a field full of tall weeds. He looked for it for ten minutes, then gave up. What happened to the ball? It got mired in the weeds.

Jesus said, "As the weeds are pulled up and burned in the fire, so it will be at the end of the age" (Matthew 13:40).

Dale Carnegie warned, "Our fatigue is caused by worry, frustration, and resentment." In other words, we tend to get mired in the weeds. In recovery, we must never lose focus. We must keep moving forward, not sidetracked by worry, frustration, or resentment.

Day 3
Confession of a Hurricane Chaser

My story is so common among addicts. I was first exposed to "it" at a very young age. It nearly destroyed our home when I was less than two years old. Then, after a few years of serenity, it came back. The effects took a toll, but we always recovered.

Then, when I was 23 and had been married for just six months, it happened again. I remember her so clearly. She came late at night and left before morning. But I was hooked. Her name was Alicia.

Hurricane Alicia.

I have been addicted to hurricanes for as long as I can remember. I've been through a number of them: Carla, Alicia, Chantal, Jerry, Ike, Irma, Michael, and Dorian.

In 2018, I drove hundreds of miles to be near the center of Michael when he came ashore the Florida Panhandle. I recorded 138 mph winds just before my arm blew off. (The farmer who recovered it in Alabama was kind enough to send it back.)

Why do I like hurricanes? One reason—I'm a man. Men are risk-takers, by nature. For some, that means surfing, jumping out of planes, starting a business, climbing mountains, or eating chili at the local diner.

And for others, it means viewing porn or surfing dating sites. It's a rush that, if left unchecked, leads to real trouble.

The answer is not to quit being a man. The answer is to put guardrails in place to limit the risks. And turn off the Weather Channel during hurricane season.

"Run from anything that stimulates youthful lusts" (2 Timothy 2:22).

Day 4
When in Rome

Where did we get the mantra, "When in Rome, do as the Romans do"? Here's the story.

Before Augustine traveled to Rome from Milan, he shared a personal dilemma with Ambrose. As a young priest, Augustine wanted to know what he should do about celebrating the Sabbath. Rome celebrated the Lord's Day on Sunday, while Milan celebrated on Saturday. This discrepancy confused Augustine and caused him to take up the matter with Ambrose.

The elder priest advised Augustine, "When in Rome, do as the Romans do."

That is good advice for world travelers. But it is dangerous counsel for the person seeking to live a life of integrity, sold out completely to God.

Revelation 3:16 says, "So, because you are lukewarm—neither hot nor cold—I am about to spit you out of my mouth" (Revelation 3:16).

John Stott said, "Apathy is the acceptance of the unacceptable."

So go ahead. When in Rome, do as the Romans do. But if it is true recovery that you want, don't "do" as those around you. That's what got you in this mess in the first place.

Day 5
Channel Surfing

"David sent someone to find out about her [Bathsheba]" (2 Samuel 11:3).

Before David got into trouble with Bathsheba he got into trouble with himself. At a time when other kings were off to war, David chose to stay back in his man cave.

It was just another spring night, and boredom set in. The couch made no demands and the remote fit snugly in his hand. David hit the channel button at random until an alluring flicker caught his eye. Reverse. Stop. Pause. He zoomed in to watch a tantalizing scene—an intimate candlelit spa. He could almost smell the candle wax and bath oil. Although the cool evening air caused a slight haze to rise from the water, the bather's physical attributes were unmistakable.

Long before channel surfing, King David knew about channel surfing. Bored, he became curious. Curious, he became enticed. Enticed, he became trapped. Then, within minutes, it seemed like hours. It was too late. The sin had been committed.

David got into trouble because he didn't get into anything else.

Anne Baxter said, "Idleness is a constant sin, and labor is a duty. Idleness is the devil's home for temptation and for unprofitable, distracting musings; while labor profits others and ourselves."

Day 6
No Snacking

Susan spent hours preparing a great meal for her husband. When he came home from work, everything was set—the table, candles, and most of all, the meticulously planned meal. Sadly, it didn't take long for Susan to notice her husband had little appetite. What had happened? Before he left work, he snacked on some cookies prepared by someone at the office.

Women can tell when their husbands have been snacking, by their loss of appetite. Similarly, when a man is viewing porn or "snacking" on some other sexual images, he loses his appetite for normal sex.

Robert Weiss, founder of The Sexual Recovery Institute, writes that casual sex "may well cause you to experience shame, depression, lowered self-esteem, and the like."

One study found that 70 percent of married men engage in pornography each year, and that the most common result is marital dissatisfaction.

Nowhere has this verse been validated more completely than within the relationship of marriage: "Your sin will find you out" (Numbers 32:23).

Guys, God created you for sex—with your wife. You will find a satisfaction in the marriage bed that cannot be found anywhere else, no matter how much snacking you do.

Day 7
Jealousy

In the Scripture, King Saul lost the throne when he saw David rising higher and gaining more influence than him. Instead of celebrating David's success, he became jealous. When people started singing, "Saul has defeated thousands," he was happy. "People are celebrating me. I've done something great!" he thought. But then the song continued, "And David has defeated tens of thousands" (1 Samuel 18:7).

Saul couldn't handle anybody being in front of him. He didn't realize they weren't in the same race. He wasn't competing with David. If Saul had been happy for David, he wouldn't have missed his destiny.

Marilyn Monroe said, "Success makes so many people hate you. I wish it wasn't that way. It would be wonderful to enjoy success without seeing envy in the eyes of those around you."

In her article, *It's a Sickness: 5 Reasons Why Jealousy Is Like Swallowing Poison*, Michele Chevrier writes, "Jealousy accomplishes the one thing nothing else can do. It guarantees that you will be the only one suffering."

Jealousy is the enemy of sobriety. Jealousy says, "I wish I had as much sobriety as Jeff does. If my wife understood me the way Steve's wife understands him, I could stay sober. If I had the kind of money Robert has, I'd be sober, too."

You need to learn this truth: the other guy isn't your competition. You are. The other guy's success doesn't make you a failure any more than his failure makes you a success.

Week 21
Honesty

"Being honest may not get you a lot of friends,

but it'll always get you the right ones."

- John Lennon

THIS WEEK'S EXERCISE
Do a FASTT Check-In

To get well, you must get honest. And to stay well, you have to stay honest. For couples who have completed a clinical disclosure, they often receive materials for follow-up. These materials usually include instructions for the couple to engage in frequent "FASTT Check-Ins." These are times when the addict communicates the status of his recovery to his wife.

The FASTT Check-In is readily available online. And while it is designed for married couples in recovery, the principles of honesty and openness are helpful for single men (or women), and as a tool to express one's progress to his sponsor or trusted accountability partner.

For this exercise, identify the person with whom you will check in. Then set up a time to meet with this person. (If you are married, this person can be your spouse.)

Follow the following formula in checking in. Remember, for this to be effective, you must be completely honest.

Feelings: What are you feeling? If there are multiple feelings, state each one.

Activities: What activities are you engaging in an effort to remain sober?

Sobriety/Slip: Express the status of your sobriety or acknowledge a recent slip.

Threats: What are the greatest threats to your sobriety this week?

Tools: What tools will you use to stay sober in the coming days?

Day 1
Getting Honest

Americans lie—a lot. *USA Today* recently cited statistics from a book, *The Day America Told the Truth*. They reported that 91% of Americans lie routinely. Specifically, 36% tell "big lies," 86% lie to their parents, 75% to their friends, 73% to their siblings, and 69% to their spouse.

What are we lying about? Eighty-one percent lie about their feelings, 43% about their income, and 40% lie about sex.

Solomon said, "The Lord hates a lying tongue" (Proverbs 6:17).

Guess who else hates "a lying tongue"? Your wife or husband. Recovery taught me something that decades of marriage never did. My wife values honesty more than anything. That's why it was so important for me to give a full disclosure of my past, accompanied with a polygraph—not just once, but several times.

William Shakespeare wrote, "Honesty is the best policy. If I lose my honor, I lose myself." One of the first things you must do to get sober is to get honest—with yourself, your spouse, and your God. Until you get completely honest, you will lose your sobriety. Worse yet, you will lose yourself.

Day 2
God's Greatest Wrath

That great philosopher Groucho Marx said, "The secret of life is honesty and fair dealing. If you can fake that, you've got it made!"

Groucho was right about one thing—the value of honesty. Unfortunately, it can't be faked. And God has a high regard for honesty.

The old prophet made God's feelings on the matter pretty clear. "Everyone who swears falsely will be banished" (Zechariah 5:3).

Don't miss the form of judgment reserved for the sin of dishonesty. God said the person will be "banished." God's greatest wrath is not functional—what he does to us. It is relational—what it does to our walk with Him.

Said another way, God's greatest judgment is not what he takes away from us, but what he takes us away from. When we are dishonest—and this is the struggle of every addict—we put in jeopardy the intimacy of our spiritual walks.

It's bad enough to lose custody of our eyes, to engage in fantasy, or worse, to slip or relapse. But to cover it up is an act of dishonesty. And this brings the gravest of judgment.

Day 3
Watermelons

The poorly paid pastor grew watermelons to supplement his income. He was doing well until he discovered several melons were stolen one night. The next night, he watched from a distance and discovered the problem. Some kids were sneaking in late at night and eating his watermelons. There were too many of them to confront, so he came up with a clever idea.

The next day, he posted a sign at the entrance to the field. It read, "Warning! One of these watermelons has been injected with cyanide."

The next day, he went out to see if the sign had worked. No watermelons had been taken, but he saw that the kids had posted their own sign, next to his. Their sign read, "Now there are two!"

American songwriter and rapper Lauren Hill said, "Reality is easy. It's deception that's the hard work."

Many of us have lived our entire lives mastering the art of deception. Like the pastor in our story, we think that if we can deceive others more successfully, we can avoid facing the real problem.

Solomon grew up hearing the stories of his own father's deceptive past. Perhaps that inspired him when he wrote, "Whoever walks in integrity walks securely, but whoever takes crooked paths will be found out" (Proverbs 10:9).

Day 4
What Women Want Most

After 37 years of marriage I have finally concluded that women are really into honesty. And that makes them incompatible with sex addicts. Dr. Milton Magness is right: "Sex addicts are world-class liars."

Most addicts think their behavior—once discovered—will be the most painful moment for their wives. And they are wrong.

Dr. Jenna Riemersma says, "For ten out of ten spouses, the lying is worse than the disclosure."

This is why our ministry is a huge proponent of using polygraphs with full disclosures. I have yet to meet the man who—under the threat of *not doing a polygraph*—became more forthcoming in describing his past behaviors. By not demanding a polygraph, the spouse (and therapist) is trusting a world-class liar to suddenly become 100 percent honest in communicating the worst behaviors he has ever committed.

As his behaviors warrant his wife's trust, this will change. If you are the wounded spouse, give yourself some space to heal. If you are the wounding spouse, give your spouse all she needs to heal. Start with this—"Let he who lied, lie no more" (Ephesians 4:25).

Day 5
Predicting Your Long-Term Sobriety

How far will you go in your sobriety? Will you find solid recovery for a lifetime? There is a way to measure such things. It's called *honesty*. Only those who are completely honest remain on track.

Professors James Kouzes and Barry Posner have spent more than 30 years surveying leaders in virtually every type of organization. They ask, "What values, personal traits, or characteristics do you look for and admire the most in a leader?"

Over these years, Kouzes and Posner have administered a survey questionnaire called *Characteristics of Admired Leaders* to more than 75,000 people on six continents. They report, "The results have been striking in their regularity over the years, and they do not vary by demographical, organizational, or cultural differences."

What is the quality that consistently tops the list?

Honesty.

The same is true in recovery. Until you come clean—completely clean—and are 100 percent known, you will be stuck on an island without a way off.

Wise Solomon said it like this: "Better the poor whose walk is blameless than a fool whose walk is perverse" (Proverbs 19:1).

Day 6
Gehazi's Fatal Mistake

2 Kings 5 tells the story of a man named Gehazi. He was an attendant of the prophet Elisha, who witnessed the miraculous healing of Naaman, the former leper. Gehazi followed Naaman out of town. When he caught up to Naaman, he told

him a huge lie. He said that Elisha had sent him to Naaman to request 200 pounds of silver (5:22).

When he returned home with the loot, Elisha asked where he had been, and Gehazi told another lie. "I didn't go anywhere" (5:25).

Gehazi was then struck with the same disease of leprosy from which Naaman had been healed.

Before he was inflicted with leprosy, Gehazi was inflicted with two fatal diseases that were much worse. First, he was consumed with greed, which Dr. Leon Seltzer calls "the ultimate addiction."

But Gehazi's troubles were compounded by his other fatal flaw—dishonesty. Notice, he was not stricken with leprosy because of his greed, but following the cover-up.

As bad as greed is—or any other addiction—it is never as fatal as the cover-up. Many a sex addict has done what Gehazi did. They did something inappropriate, then they lied about where they had been.

Day 7
Take a Chance

Breaking free from bondage and into the light is a risk worth taking. In fact, every great achievement in life involves risk.

Denis Waitley said, "Life is inherently risky. There is only one big risk you should avoid at all costs—the risk of doing nothing."

Solomon put it in agricultural terms. "He who observes the wind will not sow, and he who regards the clouds will not reap" (Ecclesiastes 11:4).

Recovering alcoholics are familiar with this line from the AA "Big Book": "Those events that once made me feel ashamed and disgraced now allow me to share with others how to become a useful member of the human race" (p. 492).

Becoming a "useful member of the human race" is reserved for those willing to take the risks of recovery: being known, transparency, and the big one—total honesty. But until you take that risk, you cannot be well.

In 2004, Kelly Clarkson recorded the hit song, *Breakaway*. Among the lyrics: "Take a chance, make a change, and break away. Out of darkness and into the sun. But I won't forget all the ones that I love. I'll take a risk."

Make that your song today. Take a chance. Make a change. Break away.

Week 22
Relapse

"Recovery is an acceptance that your life is in shambles, and you have to change it."

\- Jamie Lee Curtis

THIS WEEK'S EXERCISE
Avoid Relapse

Relapse doesn't just happen. It is the culmination of missed meetings, missed calls, and missed opportunities. And even then, relapse follows a predictable pattern.

1. We think it.
2. We plan it.
3. We do it.
4. We hate it.
5. We cover it.
6. We do it again.

The problem is really not the "do it again" phase. By the time we have thought about it and planned it, it's pretty much over. Relapse always happens in the brain before it is carried out by the body. We have sex with the wrong person in our head before we ever have sex with them in our bed.

Your job is to identify the repeated thought patterns and activities that have led to most of your relapses. And as a sex addict, you have plenty of material to work with. In order to stop the next relapse before it happens, you have to see it coming.

Here's your exercise. If you do relapse in the future, what are the triggers, causes, or circumstances that will lead you down that path if you don't deal with them in time?

- _____
- _____
- _____
- _____
- _____

Day 1
The Three Stages of Relapse

Studies indicate that 85% of those in recovery suffer relapse. How does this happen? I suggest that relapse is not some "I didn't see that coming" kind of thing. Relapse always follows a predictable pattern.

Stage 1—Emotional Relapse. The addict allows her mind to focus on the temporary pleasures of her addiction. Warning signs are isolation, not going to meetings, relaxed boundaries, and denial.

Stage 2—Mental Relapse. The addict goes from missing the pleasures of her disease to considering ways to re-engage the behaviors. Warning signs are deep cravings, euphoric recall, fantasy, minimizing consequences, and bargaining with oneself.

Stage 3—Physical Relapse. This final phase is the acting out phase. The addict returns to her destructive habits. Always, the addict bargains with herself that she will do this just once. But she discovers that she has crossed the line that Dr. S.M. Melemis calls "the point of no return."

Here's the lesson. Relapse doesn't "just happen." It is a predictable process. And that's good, because this means you can see it coming. The answer? When you find yourself slipping into Stage 1 (Emotional Relapse) step up your recovery work—immediately!

Any of us is susceptible to relapse. Take this verse to heart: "Let him who thinks he stands take heed, lest he fall" (1 Corinthians 10:12).

Day 2
#1 Cause of Relapse

The Promises Treatment Center has identified seven leading signs of a relapse on sobriety. Topping the list is this—letting up on new habits.

There is no silver bullet for recovery. It is all about doing the work, day in and day out.

There's an old joke about the farmer who was struggling to produce a good crop. He prayed, and God wrote two letters across the sky: "PC." The man assumed God was saying, "Preach Christ," so he built a pulpit at his farm and began preaching to all who came his way. When his crop continued to fail, he sought God again. He said, "I preached Christ! What more do you want me to do?"

God replied, "By 'PC,' I didn't mean to 'Preach Christ.' I was telling you to 'Plant corn.'"

The man closest to Jesus wrote, "Watch out that you do not lose what you have worked so hard to achieve. Be diligent, so you may receive your full reward" (2 John 8).

In one week, I had two friends who both lost their sobriety after three years. They both had one thing in common—they let up on their daily disciplines.

Recovery is hard work, day in and day out. It's about establishing new habits, and then sticking to the plan every day for the rest of your life.

Day 3
The Power of a Bad Day

Past victories are no guarantee of future success.

Toward the end of Noah's amazing life we read this sad account. "Noah drank some wine and became drunk and lay uncovered inside his tent. Ham saw his father naked and told his two brothers outside. But Shem and Japheth took a garment and laid it across their shoulders; then they walked in backward and covered their father's naked body. Their faces were turned the other way so that they would not see their father naked" (Genesis 9:21-23).

Much of what Noah had accomplished in his first 600 years was washed away by one bad night. What went wrong?

Past victories are no guarantee of future success.

The following enjoyed great success early in life, only to die broke: Vincent van Gogh, Joe Louis, Sammy Davis, Jr., Oscar Wilde, Edgar Allan Poe, and Judy Garland.

History is full of examples of celebrity icons who fell from grace. O.J. Simpson and Bill Cosby come to mind.

Noah was a man of eminent distinction. But one bad day of self-indulgence put images into the minds of his sons that they would never forget. The lesson? Celebrate your past victories. But stay humble, because past victories are no guarantee of future success.

Day 4
Fighting Back

When facing temptations, you will be attacked daily. It never stops. The enemy will come at you in every way that he can and wherever he sees an opening. That is why you must be prepared to fight back, with all the tools available.

Paul said it like this: "Put on the full armor of God, so that you can take your stand against the devil's schemes" (Ephesians 6:11).

Relapse isn't the road of least *resistance* as much as it is the road of least *persistence*. True, lasting recovery is reserved for those willing to stay in the battle and fight every day for the rest of their lives.

Early in my recovery, I had a slip. But I kept going to meetings. Then I had another slip. So I got a sponsor. And then another slip. I started working the Steps. Still another slip. I added another meeting each week.

Then I collected my first chip. I had been sober for 30 days. Then two months. Eventually, six months, then a year, two years, and eventually five years.

What brought the breakthrough? It is simple. When my addiction hit, I hit back—harder. And to this day, I never quit punching.

Day 5
A New Set of Eyes

Basketball hall-of-famer John Wooden said, "It's what you do after you know it all that counts."

My Westie checks off all the boxes—loyal, smart, cute, fun, energetic, and—obstinate. I think that's why we get along so well. We share all six qualities in common. Well, at least we are both obstinate.

People come by this condition naturally. (I'm not sure why my dog is that way.) We always think we are right. We dig in our heels. We fight for a position, not because we really believe it, but because we've already said it. It's not that it's the right idea, but that it's our idea.

God says, "I will instruct you and show you the way to go; with my eye on you, I will give counsel. Do not be like a horse or mule, without understanding, that must be controlled with bit and bridle or else it will not come near you" (Psalm 32:8-9).

If you are to find your way out of your addiction, you'll need a different set of eyes than the pair that got you into your addiction in the first place. You need

God's counsel and His direction. The good news is that He stands ready to give you both.

Day 6
Avoid Relapse: A Three-Step Plan

We will begin today's column with a sobering thought. Mike Loverde, founder of Family First Intervention, says that of those who complete a substance abuse rehab program, 70-90% will relapse. The Bible says, "As a dog returns to its vomit, so a fool returns to his folly" (Proverbs 26:11).

Relapse is common, but it is a bump in the road, not a dead end.

Dr. David Sack wrote, in *Why Relapse Isn't a Sign of Failure*, "Study after study shows the first 90 days in recovery are when the greatest percentage of relapse occurs."

Why is relapse so common during the first 90 days of sobriety? The brain is still rewiring, new habits are still being formed, and acting out memories are still fresh.

I am so convinced that the first 90 days are critical that I wrote **A 90-Day Recovery Guide**. In the book, I assert, "Although 90 days of sobriety cannot guarantee a lifetime of recovery, it is the start you so desperately need."

What follows your first 90 days will largely depend on the habits you establish within those 90 days. In my book, I suggest the following three tools as essential ingredients to avoiding relapse: (a) a disciplined plan, (b) a spiritual program, and (c) a personal coach.

The good news is that relapse doesn't have to be fatal. But the better news is that it doesn't have to happen at all.

Day 7
Good Behavior Is Not Enough

When recovery only involves changes in behavior rather than changes of the heart, it does not last. Case in point—the people in Malachi's time.

The last book of the Old Testament contains the message of a Jewish prophet named Malachi. He was writing to the people of Judah, the Southern Kingdom. It was God's final word before the coming of Christ 400 years later. Malachi's message came on the heels of two significant outward victories—the building of the Temple and the rebuilding of the walls around Jerusalem, under the leadership of Nehemiah.

Their success as a nation led to complacency, which led to relapse into their old ways. God's response: "I am the Lord, and I do not change. That is why you descendants of Jacob are not already destroyed" (Malachi 3:6).

To avoid relapse, you must remain diligent. Dr. Milton Magness asserts, in *Real Hope, True Freedom*, "Each time a person resists the urge to act out, his recovery gets stronger, and so will yours."

Like Judah, you may have achieved success by all outward appearances. To others, your sobriety appears secure. But don't ignore the heart. That's where relapse always begins.

Week 23
Surrender

"God is ready to assume full responsibility
for the life wholly yielded to him."

- Andrew Murray

THIS WEEK'S EXERCISE
Plan a Sweet Surrender

Step 3 says, "We made a decision to turn our wills and our lives over to the care of God as we understood God." That is a decision we all must make—every day.

But deciding to surrender to God is not the same thing as actually surrendering to God. This week, you will take the sweet step of surrender. You will read about surrender in this week's devotions. But first, set aside a few minutes for this powerful exercise.

Below, make a list of all the things in your life that you need to let go of, that you need to surrender to God. Then write each of them on a separate scrap of paper. It is best to do this in several settings, as you will think of new areas to surrender each time you focus on this. Once you feel comfortable that you have written down everything that needs to be surrendered, move to the most important part of the exercise.

Take those scraps of paper and find a place of solitude. Then get down on your knees and surrender each of these parts of your life to God. As you release each one, place that scrap of paper next to you. When you are finished, pick up those papers and discard them. Put them in a trash can where you can never go back and retrieve them.

Things I will surrender to God:

- _____
- _____
- _____
- _____
- _____
- _____
- _____

Where I will go to surrender these to God: _____

Date I will surrender these things: _____

Day 1
The Meaning of Surrender

Oscar Wilde wrote, "Everything in the world is about sex except sex. Sex is about power."

Research confirms this thesis. Sex is about power. And addicts can never get enough. Many of us can identify with the line in *Top Gun*. We have an incredible "need for speed."

This speed comes in many forms—with sex at the top of the list. Like those who struggle with substances, impulse control disorders, or behavioral addictions, sexual addicts find themselves with ever-growing passions and ever-diminishing satisfaction.

This is what makes recovery so hard for so many. We want sobriety, but we also want power. We want to be in control. But we can't have both. Recovery is absolutely rooted in surrender.

How do we find victory? James offers clear insight. "Submit yourselves therefore to God. Resist the devil, and he will flee from you" (James 4:7).

Oswald Chambers was right: "If you have only come as far as asking God for things, you have never come to understand the meaning of surrender."

Day 2
Apollo 13

The day was Monday, April 13, 1970. The crew of Apollo 13 found themselves marooned 200,000 miles from Earth. During a routine maintenance task, one of the spacecraft's four oxygen tanks exploded. For the next four days, astronauts Jim Lovell, Jack Swigert, and Fred Haise worked against all odds to bring their wounded ship back to Earth.

People around the world prayed for the trio's safe return. Each time the engineers at NASA solved one problem, another took its place. But a little faith and a lot of sweat eventually worked wonders. After four long days, Apollo 13's parachutes opened. The craft lowered safely into the Pacific Ocean.

Perhaps your "spaceship" is spiraling out of control. As with Apollo 13, the answer is not hard work or prayer. The answer is hard work and prayer.

St. Augustine said, "Pray as though everything depends on God, then work as though everything depends on you."

Solomon said it like this: "Commit to the Lord whatever you do, and he will establish your plans" (Proverbs 16:3).

You may have battled porn and sex addiction for years. Don't give up! If you work hard and pray hard, your ship can still have a safe landing.

If your spacecraft is out of control, do what only you can do. Then trust God to do what only he can do.

Day 3
Escape

Have you heard of a book called *The Worst Case Survival Guide*? The author puts meticulous research to work, providing us a way out of the most common dilemmas in which we might find ourselves. Chapters include "How to escape from a sinking car," "How to jump from a building into a dumpster," and "How to escape from a bear."

Missing are the chapters I need: "How to find your way home when Google Maps are down," "How to reset the clock on the microwave," and "How to restart your jet ski when it dies 300 yards from the beach and you see a four-foot long shark three feet from the ski."

How about this one: "How to escape the clutches of a personal addiction."

Actually, there already is a Survival Guide for that one. It is the same Guide that tells us how the Israelites escaped the Egyptian army, how Daniel escaped the lion's den, and how Peter escaped his prison cell.

In the darkness of the night, God opened the cell for which Peter had no key. "Then Peter came to himself and said, 'Now I know without a doubt that the Lord has sent his angel and rescued me from Herod's clutches'" (Acts 12:11).

You can escape the prison of your addiction. The key that unlocks the door is called surrender—it's about letting God do for you what you cannot do for yourself. As for jumping into a dumpster—well, you're on your own with that one.

Day 4
Princess Diana

Proverbs 24:16 says, "For though the righteous fall seven times, they rise again, but the wicked stumble when calamity strikes."

Few people in modern history epitomize the power of overcoming as did Princess Diana. Marrying into the Royal Family gave her a platform of influence known to a precious few. But her divorce from Prince Charles in 1996 did not change that. Such was her impact through her support of AIDS research, leprosy cures, and a ban on land mines that when Diana died in 1997 at the age of 36, her funeral was carried in 44 languages and viewed by 2.5 billion people.

There's a line in *Braveheart*, the 1995 war film about William Wallace. Wallace was a 13th century Scottish warrior who led the Scots in the First War of Scottish Independence against King Edward I of England. Played by Mel Gibson, Wallace said, "Every man dies, but not every man really lives."

Addiction brings a form of death—to the addict, his reputation, his family. Upon his discovery, his habit may end the life he once knew. But there is still time to pick up the pieces and really live, perhaps for the first time.

The question is not whether you have fallen. You have. We all have. The question is what you will do next. It's what comes after you fall that will determine your ultimate destiny.

Day 5
The Power of One

It is one of the most quoted verses in the Bible. "I can do all things through Christ who strengthens me" (Philippians 4:13).

One plus God equals enough. Dalai Lama said, "If you think you are too small to make a difference, try sleeping with a mosquito."

You can make a difference—on your own. The same is true of recovery. While it is always recommended that you see a therapist, get to a 12-Step group, and build accountability among a small group of same-sex men or women in recovery, you can find recovery—even if no one else stands beside you to help.

How does this work? B.J. Gallagher and Steve Ruttenberg answer that question in *The Power of One*, in which they outline dozens of examples of how one person made a huge difference. They recommend a four-step process: (a) believe, (b) act, (c) lead, (d) transform.

It starts with *believe*. If you believe in Christ as your Higher Power, and then in yourself, you can overcome temptation, pain, and addictions—of all types.

Day 6
Just One Stomach Flu Away

There's a line in the 2006 movie, *The Devil Wears Prada*. Emily Charlton said, "I'm just one stomach flu away from my goal weight."

While this is a statement about body image and self-perception, the line also speaks to addiction. Let me explain.

Sometimes, we have to get really sick in order to get really well. It often takes an STD, loss of a job, or marital breakup to get a man's attention. Until he loses something he is not ready to gain something. Why? Because a man or woman must become desperate in order to become well.

We've heard the phrase "no pain, no gain" 1.5 zillion times. Some sources trace the origin of this truism back to the second century writings of Rabbi Ben Hei Hei. He wrote, in *The Ethics of the Fathers*, "According to the pain is the gain."

I'm not sure I've ever met a man or woman who got into successful recovery who did not first lose something and become sick over their destructive behaviors. In order to find recovery, we must embrace the ethics of Christ, who asked, "What shall it profit a man if he gains the whole world, but loses his own soul?" (Mark 8:36).

You must lose before you gain. You must hunger before you are filled. And you will probably have to suffer in some way before you will be willing to go all in with recovery.

Day 7
Step 6

Step 6 says, "We were entirely ready to have God remove all these defects of character." How do we honestly get to that point? We see an example in John 5.

There was a pool where people went, hoping to experience miraculous healing. But to receive the miracle, it was thought that they had to get to the water. One fellow, sick for 38 years, was lying by the pool. Jesus confronted him and asked if he wanted to be made well. The man responded, "I have no one to put me into the pool" (John 5:6).

This man was so crippled that he couldn't go any farther on his own. He camped as close as he could to the place where there was hope for recovery. God met him there and brought him the rest of the way.

That's how recovery works. You go as far as you can, but you still come up short. Then, when you are *entirely ready*, God stands in, fully prepared to carry you the rest of the way.

Dwight L. Moody used to say, at the end of his messages, "Now it's time to walk forward to trust Jesus. If you can't make it all the way down to the front, just take the steps you can, and God will carry you the rest of the way."

There comes a time for each of us when we need to be carried. If you are *entirely ready*, reach out to God. Why? Because he can take you where you could otherwise never go.

Week 24
Guardrails

"Givers need to set limits because takers rarely do."

- Rachel Wolchin

THIS WEEK'S EXERCISE
Build a Guardrail

Across America, the Highway Department has erected 4,386,000 miles of guardrails along federal highways. Actually, I made that up. But here's something I didn't make up—guardrails have saved thousands of lives. If you are a newer driver, let me explain how this works. You aren't supposed to get as close as you can without going over the edge of the road. If you do that, there will eventually be an unexpected bump in the road, and you'll lose it.

In recovery, guardrails represent the steps we take to keep us from going over the edge. Curiosity says, "I wonder what is on the other side of the guardrail." Intelligence says, "Don't go there. It's just too dangerous."

We all need guardrails in order to keep our recovery in the safe zone. These will be different for each of us. What you need to do in order to stay safe may not work for me, and vice versa. And the guardrails will change, depending on where we are in our recovery. That means that this week's exercise is one you may want to revisit in a few months.

Here we go. Pick one of the guardrails from the list below. If none of these seem to fit your personal recovery needs, identify a different guardrail. For now, just pick one, and write down your specific plan for that guardrail.

- Get on Covenant Eyes: _____

- End a toxic relationship: _____

- Go to bed earlier at night: _____

- Change your TV habits: _____

- Adjust your social media exposure: _____

- Give your spouse access to your phone: _____

- Avoid certain areas of town: _____

- Limit the cash you carry: _____

- Don't be alone with the opposite sex: _____

- Limit time on your computer: _____

- Other: _____

Day 1
Stay Off the Highway

The national highway system consists of 164,000 miles of highways. A few years ago, Beth and I were driving on one of those highways, following a conference in Colorado. It was the highest elevated highway in America, leading to a beautiful spot atop Mt. Evans. It was the perfect drive, except for one thing—no guardrails.

While there was technically no reason to stay off this particular road, what I was doing was dangerous. And it was a parable on recovery.

Paul wrote, "All things are lawful for me, but not all things are helpful" (2 Corinthians 6:12). In other words, there are things we can do that are not bad, but they are dangerous.

I find great truth in the words of one of my favorite actors, Michael J. Fox. "Life is good, and there's no reason to think it won't be—right up until the moment when everything explodes into a fireball of tiny, unrecognizable fragments, or it all goes skidding sideways, through the guardrail, over the embankment, and down the mountain."

Substitute "recovery" for "life." Your recovery is good, and there's no reason to think it won't be. But because you have no guardrails, you may find yourself "skidding sideways, over the embankment, and down the mountain."

The key to recovery is not to drive perfectly. The key is not to check off all the boxes of perfect sobriety. The key is to stay off dangerous roads.

Day 2
It Only Takes an Hour

I recently heard about a pastor who, in five minutes, lost his entire reputation. It doesn't take long. Saul, the first king of Israel, is a perfect example. Though a mighty warrior and strong leader, he lost it all—in one hour.

Israel was at war with the Philistines. Things looked bleak. "Saul stayed at Gilgal, and his men were trembling with fear" (1 Samuel 13:7). Samuel had instructed the king to wait until he arrived, and then he would make a burnt offering to the Lord. But after seven days, Saul grew impatient. His anxiety overtook his better judgment, so he made the offering himself, in violation of the law and Samuel's commands. When he arrived, Samuel told Saul that his sin would have consequences. "Your kingdom must end" (13:13).

If Saul had waited another hour, he would have kept his kingdom. But like many of us, he lost it all—in order to control things himself—for just one hour.

When the urge to act out hits, know that this will pass. It always does. When the urge hits, only focus on the next hour. Pray. Make a call. Read Scripture. Take a walk. If you can make it for an hour, you can make it!

You make your decisions, then your decisions make you. Be alert. Be on guard. All the recovery you have built up over the past several months or years can come crashing down—in less than an hour.

Day 3
Close the Window

It happened on April 17, 1790. Ben Franklin died from sitting in front of his window. Here's what happened. Franklin was a big believer in fresh air. So every night, he slept with the window open. He wrote, "I rise every morning and sit near the window in my chamber without any clothes, regardless of the season."

April of 1790 started like any other time in the 84-year-old's life. But this time, Franklin developed an abscess in his lungs, which his doctors attributed to his many hours sitting naked in front of an open window. The abscess burst on April 17, and he died a few hours later.

Many of us suffer from open windows. We open the window to temptation— just a little—and we are okay. Until we're not.

Peter warned, "Keep away from worldly desires that wage war against your very souls" (1 Peter 2:11).

Maintaining sobriety is a war. It will probably be the most difficult battle you ever face. One of the keys to victory is to keep the window of temptation nailed shut. Don't even crack the window a little. This may mean you need to avoid certain places, television shows, or toxic relationships. If you allow the window of temptation to remain open, you will soon find yourself like Ben Franklin—naked and helpless.

It's time to shut the window.

Day 4
Waterloo

The Battle of Waterloo was fought on June 18, 1815, near the city of Waterloo in present day Belgium. All of England knew that the Duke of Wellington was leading the British forces against the French Emperor, Napoleon Bonaparte, in this epic battle. A ship signaled news of the outcome of the battle to a man on top of Winchester Cathedral. The message consisted of three words: "Wellington defeated Napoleon."

But the fog rolled in before the man at the Cathedral saw the third word. So the message that went out across England was, "Wellington defeated." The British thought they had lost the decisive battle, which they had actually won.

Sometimes we get mixed messages. In recovery, we often feel defeated—until we realize this battle is not our own. Our Higher Power has already defeated the enemy. We don't live *for* that victory, but *from* it.

Sun Tzu had it right: "The supreme art of war is to subdue the enemy without fighting."

Because the battle has already been won, we can say, "Give glory to him who is able to keep you from falling and to present you before his glorious presence without fault and with joy" (Jude 24).

Yes, the enemy is strong. But you must hear the full message. The enemy was defeated.

Claim the victory that has been secured on the cross.

Day 5
Standing Aloof

How does a person fall?

The Old Testament prophet warned, "On the day you stood aloof, you too were as one of them" (Obadiah 11).

Edmund Burke said it like this: "The only thing necessary for the triumph of evil is for good men to do nothing."

On a national level, this happens one generation at a time. There is this phenomenon called the "third generation principle." It states that when a generation produces significant change (such as the Great Generation), the generation which follows will move toward entrenchment. And the third generation will bring about decline.

The same thing happens in our individual lives. We naturally devolve from active production to complacency to decline. And it all starts with what Obadiah called standing "aloof."

When you are confronted with temptation, trauma, and trouble, you have three choices: (a) stand strong, (b) stand weak, or (c) stand aloof. It's that third one that becomes the unseen trap.

Day 6
Safety Plan

Mark and Debra Laaser wrote *The Seven Desires of Every Heart*. They identify the first desire as the need to feel safe.

Perhaps you are a betrayed spouse, and you just don't feel safe right now. This is actually an issue of the brain.

You were created with a sympathetic nervous system. This is the "gas" that ignites behavioral responses to traumatic events. The SNS will elicit one of two unintended reactions to fear. All mammals have the SNS.

For example, when you approach a frog sitting on a rock, his SNS will kick in a "flight" response, causing him to leap into the lake. But when you approach a wild dog, his SNS may elicit a "fight" response, meaning that approaching this dog may be the last decision you will make in this life.

As humans, we have automatic responses to outward threats and traumatic memories. Therefore, when your spouse has been with prostitutes, engaged in frequent porn, or indulged in other illicit behaviors, this will bring an emotional response that is reactive, not cognitive. It comes from your sympathetic nervous system.

In short, if your spouse has done things that make you feel unsafe, that is on him. You need to formulate a long-term safety plan that makes you feel safe, whether it makes sense to your partner or not.

God wants you to feel safe. That's why we read, "He who dwells in the shelter of the Most High will abide in the shadow of the Almighty" (Psalm 91:1).

Day 7
When She Jumps in Your Car

In the SA "white book," there is the story of a seminary student who was working in a local church. His sex addiction was destroying his marriage and his ministry. After twelve years of living in his addiction, he left all behind, in search of hope and freedom. Then, he writes, "One night, out of nowhere, a prostitute jumped into my car."

The prostitute jumping into the car is a metaphor with which every addict can identify. This "prostitute" represents all kinds of sexual sin. For that matter, she represents all kinds of sin—period.

Every Christ-follower knows what it is to have temptation "jump into his car." Sometimes, this "prostitute" jumps in your car without an invitation. So what is the answer? I propose five solutions.

1. Lock the doors to your car. Be diligent. Put in place every protection possible to keep the "prostitute" out.
2. Avoid certain neighborhoods. Avoid the part of town where "prostitutes" can be found. Just don't go there. Don't put yourself in vulnerable situations.
3. Keep your car moving. No one can jump into a moving car. It is when you slow down to look around, when you take your eyes off the road, that you get into trouble.
4. Don't travel alone. The "prostitute" is less likely to jump into your car if you have someone with you. It's called accountability. We all need it.
5. Just say no. When all else fails, say no. You don't have to open the door. Every time you commit sexual (or any other) sin, it is a choice of the moment. Just say no.

"Each person is tempted when they are dragged away by their own evil desire and enticed" (James 1:14). Most of the time, you can avoid the temptations that kill and destroy. And when that temptation does "jump in" uninvited, remember, there is always a way out.

Week 25
Isolation

*"A person is a person through other persons;
you can't be human in isolation; you
are human only in relationships."*

\- Desmond Tutu

THIS WEEK'S EXERCISE
Don't Isolate

Isolation is not your friend. While it is healthy to schedule "alone" times, you cannot maintain sobriety apart from the fellowship of others. You need to be a part of a recovery group, a Bible study small group, and other groups. You were created to have a personal relationship with God, but not a private relationship with God. You need others, and others need you.

In additional to connecting with a group, you need a mentor—someone with more sobriety than you have. Scripture is full of such examples. David/Jonathan and Paul/Timothy come to mind immediately.

So here's your task for this week. Get with someone you know, who has more sobriety than you. You can visit with them over lunch or over the phone. Maybe you can schedule time before or after a recovery meeting. It's best to meet in person, if possible.

Ask them two questions: how they got sober and how they stay sober. Then journal below, reflecting on what you learn.

Person you will meet with: _____

When you will meet: _____

How they got sober: _____

_____

_____

_____

_____

_____

How they stay sober: _____

_____

_____

_____

_____

Day 1
Isolation

Pitcairn Island is one of the most remote places on earth. Set in the Pacific Ocean, it is home to just 50 residents, and for good reason—you can't get there. You must fly to Tahiti and then sail for 1,200 miles. Then you transfer to a ruby dinghy, take your climbing gear and eventually scale the 900-foot rock cliffs to the tiny village.

Pitcairn Island is a metaphor on loneliness and isolation. Pitcairn Island is a metaphor on addiction.

Solomon wrote, "Whoever isolates himself seeks his own desire; he rejects sound judgment" (Proverbs 18:1).

Addicts come in all shapes and sizes. Addiction knows no color or creed, race or religion. But if you look hard enough and long enough into every addict's past you will find the same thing.

Isolation.

Hear the words of John Lennon's hit song from 1970: *"People say we've got it made. Don't they know we're so afraid? We're afraid to be alone. Everybody got to have a home."*

The facts are these: Nobody has it made, we're all afraid, we don't want to be alone, and we've all got to have a home.

Here's the thing. Isolation is not a condition as much as it is a choice. So join the family of God, get in a support group, and get outside yourself. Why? Because if you don't defeat the demon of isolation, the demon of isolation will defeat you.

Join a group. Get in a church. Make some new friends. That is the key to sanity, hope, and freedom.

Day 2
All for One, One for All

John Dickerson, a Founding Father of the United States, spoke to the events of his day with the famous words, "United we stand, divided we fall," published in the *Boston Gazette* in July 1768.

French author Alexandre Dumas picked up on this theme in writing his most famous novel, *The Three Musketeers*, in 1844. The book recounts the adventures of a young man named Charles de Batz de Castelmore d'Artagnan, who left home to serve Louis XIV as captain of the Musketeers from 1632 to 1673. In a pact to remain loyal to one another through thick and thin, d'Artagnan and his fellow Musketeers adopted the following as their motto for life:

"All for one and one for all; united we stand, divided we fall."

The three Musketeers might have been the first recovery group. This kind of unity and mutual support is critical to lasting sobriety and daily victory. As John Maxwell says, "None of us is as strong as all of us."

Paul said it like this: "I appeal to you, brothers and sisters, in the name of our Lord Jesus Christ, that all of you agree with one another in what you say and that there be no divisions among you, but that you be perfectly united in mind and thought" (1 Corinthians 1:10).

The road to recovery is long and winding, with many hills and valleys, passing through treacherous lands unseen until they are conquered. It is foolish to tread such a road by oneself. You need to join with others for the walk.

Say it with me: *"All for one and one for all; united we stand, divided we fall."* Identify a small recovery group and join them for the journey.

Day 3
All Alone

Dr. Shahram Heshmat wrote an excellent article, *Addiction as a Disease of Isolation*. He makes the case for isolation as a leading contributor to addiction.

He writes, "Since insecurely attached individuals doubt the availability and support of others, they use other tactics to mitigate and control negative affect. One compensatory strategy is attachment to non-human targets (for example, objects and materialism). In other words, they substitute relationships with objects for relationships with people."

Heshmat is suggesting that in our addiction we avoid personal connections. We isolate. And that never ends well. Consider the prophet Elijah, for example.

"The Israelites have rejected your covenant, torn down your altars, and put your prophets to death with the sword. I am the only one left, and now they are trying to kill me, too" (1 Kings 19:10).

Elijah actually had 7,000 others ready to stand by his side. But in the face of difficulty, he retreated into isolation and depression. The fact is, isolation is a choice. You are only alone if you choose to be. Be aware—your isolation feeds your addiction. And that never ends well.

Dr. Heshmat is right. Sex addicts treat women as objects in order to avoid personal connections. That leads to isolation, and that never ends well.

Day 4
Allota Warmheart

The year was 1985. When Beth and I stepped out of the elevator at the Fairmont Hotel in San Francisco, we were greeted by the sound of clicking cameras. Why? Because Elizabeth Taylor was staying at the same hotel. And she was expected to come down the same elevator to the lobby below. The media knew she was there because the woman who appeared on the cover of *Life Magazine* more than any other person always traveled under her own name.

Contrast that with Allota Warmheart. Allota would be as famous to her generation as Elizabeth Taylor was to hers. But unlike Ms. Taylor, Allota doesn't travel under her real name, because she prefers her anonymity.

The Bible says, "I praise you because I am fearfully and wonderfully made; your works are wonderful, I know that full well" (Psalm 139:14).

Tim Keller has written, "To be loved but not known is comforting but superficial. To be known and not loved is our greatest fear. But to be fully known and truly loved is, well, a lot like being loved by God. It is what we need more than anything. It liberates us from pretense, humbles us out of our self-righteousness, and fortifies us for any difficulty life can throw at us."

There is nothing so liberating as being fully known. And as for Allota Warmheart, you may know her better as Britney Spears.

You need to be fully known—by God and someone else. So find a way to tell your story. It will bring freedom to your heart and hope to the hearts of others.

Day 5
Time to Come Out

Mike Genung has identified 11 steps to breaking free from sexual addiction, in *The Road to Grace: Finding True Freedom from the Bondage of Sexual Addiction*. He says the first step to freedom is to come out of isolation.

Isolation is depicted brilliantly in the movie *Burnt*, in which Bradley Cooper plays the role of Adam, a chef who battles a trio of addictions: women, drugs, and alcohol. Adam's road is a rocky one. On that road he learns how to ask for help and how to quit isolating from family, colleagues, and friends. He discovers the strength that comes from needing others.

If you are to get well—and stay well—you must learn the lesson that Adam learned. You cannot do this on your own. You can have recovery or isolation, but you can't have both.

The psalmist wrote, "Though my father and mother forsake me, the Lord will receive me" (Psalm 27:10).

The first relationship that breaks through the wall of isolation is a spiritual one. Whether driven to isolation by parents, family members, or friends, you don't have to stay there. When you are all alone, you are not all alone. And no matter what you have done, the Lord will receive you.

Break down the wall of isolation by connecting with God. Seek to find that connection today.

Day 6
Withdrawal

Robin Williams said, "Cocaine for me was a place to hide. Most people get hyper on coke. It slowed me down. Sometimes it made me paranoid and impotent, but mostly it just made me withdrawn."

And therein lies one of the cruel effects of addiction.

Withdrawal.

When we are active in our illicit behaviors, living a double life, we withdraw—from family, friends, and God. We live in shame and fear. We fear being found out and being fully known. And we live in guilt. "What if they knew what I was doing?" we ask. And so the cycle continues.

The pattern is predictable: (a) bad choices, (b) bad behavior, (c) guilt and shame, (d) fear, (e) withdrawal, (f) more bad choices.

There is a way out. It's called becoming desperate. And in that desperation we turn to God, but rarely before.

We are promised, "You will seek me and find me when you search for me with all your heart" (Jeremiah 29:13).

Day 7
Sticky Friends

The Bible praises the "friend who sticks closer than a brother" (Proverbs 18:24).

Since entering recovery several years ago, I have benefited greatly from education, with a Master's in Addiction Recovery (Liberty University) and the PSAP certification (Pastoral Sex Addiction Professional). But some things I've learned have come from pure experience. One of those truths is the absolute necessity of friends in order to secure recovery.

To find recovery with the help of others is difficult; to do it alone, impossible. You will need at least two or three others (same sex as you) who are on the same path that you are on, who will be on your side—no matter what.

The Bible says we need a "friend who sticks." What does this "sticky friend" look like? I suggest three things.

1. They draw near because you fell, not because you were perfect.
2. They give you their time more than their advice.
3. They are still there when nobody else is.

You need a "sticky friend." May you find one soon.

Week 26
Inventory

"There is nothing noble in being superior to your fellow men.
True nobility lies in being superior to your former self."

- Ernest Hemingway

THIS WEEK'S EXERCISE
Peel an Orange

This week's exercise will be the tastiest one you will do all year. You need to buy, steal, or borrow an orange. Once you have your orange, you can proceed with this exercise.

Okay, have your orange?

Follow these directions very carefully . . .

1. Peel your orange.
2. Eat your orange.

Hopefully, you were able to keep up. Now for the hard part. Your orange represents your life and personal recovery. Let me offer several points to this analogy.

First, what others see on the outside rarely matches what is on the inside. Think about it. If you had never seen the inside of an orange, would you have really known what it would look like once you peeled away the rind? Similarly, when others look at you, they are seeing the outside, not the inner struggles, pain, and addictions.

Second, you can't get to the good part until you peel away the cover. No one eats the rind. We peel it away, and quickly discard it. It is what we find beyond the rind that matters. Likewise, no matter how damaged or bruised we may be on the inside, it is that inside—not our outer appearance—that matters most.

Third, getting to the heart of the orange is messy. Our hands get wet and sticky. But it's worth it, because the juicy orange segments beyond the rind bring satisfaction and pleasure.

Now, let's apply the orange to your life.

1. How frustrated did you get trying to get to the "good part" of the orange? _____

_____

2. What are the layers of your life that still need to be peeled back? _____

_____

3. Are you willing to go through the messy process of peeling back your cover in order to find lasting recovery? What might that look like? _____

_____

Day 1
Unintentional Sin

Is it possible to sin—unintentionally? The Bible says yes. In the Levitical Law we read, "Say to the Israelites, 'When anyone sins unintentionally and does what is forbidden in any of the Lord's commands, he must bring a young bull to the Lord'" (Leviticus 4:2).

Let's break that down. We see two things here. First, it is possible to cross some lines, break some commands, and commit some sins—without being aware of it at the time. Second, we must own the results. The fact that their mistakes might have been unintended did not exonerate God's children from the damage caused.

You may have hurt your spouse without even knowing it. An unintended glance, viewing an old friend's Facebook page, talking to the lady at church—you did none of these things from bad motives. But given the damage you have already brought upon your marriage, these actions caused pain.

Unintended actions have unintended consequences. But these are still consequences. And the pain is real.

Blaise Pascal said, "There are only two kinds of men: the righteous who think they are sinners and the sinners who think they are righteous." We all continue to make mistakes from time to time. That's not the issue. But we must atone for those mistakes—intended or not.

You may have committed unintended sins against your husband or wife. It's time to own it and atone for what you've done.

Day 2
Take-Home Exams

Angelina Jolie said, "I don't see myself as beautiful, because I see a lot of flaws."

How do you see yourself? The old prophet wisely advised, "Now this is what the Lord Almighty says: 'Give careful thought to your ways'" (Haggai 1:5).

On the road to recovery, you must avoid two ditches. On one side of the road is the "I'm okay" ditch. We drive into this ditch when we refuse to acknowledge our struggles.

On the other side of the road is the "I'm a horrible human being" ditch. We drive into this ditch when we define ourselves by our shortcomings.

Haggai recommended driving in the middle lane. Step 4 of all 12-Step programs says it like this: "We made a searching and fearless moral inventory of ourselves."

When was the last time you did that? Recovery calls for frequent take-home exams. It calls on us to take periodic moral inventories. We cannot define ourselves by our faults, nor must we run from them. Instead, we must grow from them.

Take an honest, fearless, moral inventory of yourself. Don't define yourself by your faults and don't ignore them. Acknowledge them. Confess them. Then move on.

Day 3
Taking the 4th Step

Jason Wahler, founder of Widespread Recovery, states, "The addiction is but a symptom of a spiritual disease. The real problem is in character flaws that need to be faced and overcome. This requires one thing—total honesty."

Therein lies the rub—total honesty. This is what the 4th Step is all about. This is what recovery is all about. Most of us wished we could have avoided taking a personal inventory. It's normal to hide from personal examination. But in our hearts we knew that day would come when we would have to face the truth about ourselves.

The Bible warns of a day when no man can hide. "And I saw the dead, great and small, standing before the throne, and books were opened. Another book was opened, which is the book of life. The dead were judged according to what they had done as recorded in the books" (Revelation 20:12).

It is best to do our inventory now, so we will be ready for the big one to come. The 4th Step is just nine words: "Made a searching and fearless moral inventory of ourselves." But those are nine powerful words. To get well, you have to get honest—about your past, your struggles, and most of all, your character defects. You're going to have to come clean eventually; you might as well do it now.

If you haven't already done so, under the guidance of your sponsor, you need to work the 4th Step.

Day 4
Join the List

St. Francis of Assisi said, "If God can work through me, he can work through anyone." The great apostle Paul called himself "chief among sinners" (1 Timothy 1:15). God uses people others would discard. Consider the following list from Scripture.

- Abraham—too old
- Jeremiah—too young
- Zacchaeus—too small
- Gideon—too timid
- Disciples—too disorganized
- Noah—a drunk
- Jacob—a cheater
- David—a murderer
- Naomi—a widow
- Martha—a worrier
- Rahab—a prostitute
- Samson—a womanizer
- Elijah—suicidal
- Joseph—abused
- Job—bankrupt
- Moses—speech problem
- Samaritan woman—divorced
- Jonah—ran from God
- Peter—denied Christ

Francis was right. If God could use him, he can use anybody. I put myself at the very top of the "If God can use me" list. Now it's your turn. The fact is, God wants to use you—not despite your mistakes, but because of them. The next move is yours.

Confess your sins, then move on. God stands ready to use you now in ways you can't begin to imagine.

Day 5
Sexual Desire

We think about sex—a lot. Writing for *Psychology Today*, Dr. Brian Mustanski stated the results of an extensive study. Men think about sex 18.6 times a day, compared to 9.9 times for women.

Modern society has turned sex into something God never intended for it to be. Every day, we are bombarded with new stories about sex identity confusion, sexual predators, and sex offenders. Women (and men) are often portrayed as sexual figures in the media before they are seen as anything else.

But sex is a good thing, as created by God. Author Gary Thomas writes, "We need to look at sexual desire through the lens of creation, rather than through the lens of the fall."

John Piper said, in his message, *Why Did God Create Sexual Desire*, "God created sexual desire. That makes it good."

The same Bible that says, "For God so loved the world" (John 3:16) and "Love the Lord your God" (Deuteronomy 6:5) also says this: "Your stature is like a palm tree; your breasts are clusters of fruit. I said, 'I will climb the palm tree and take hold of its fruit'" (Song of Songs 7:7).

Sexual desire is a good thing. And sexual fulfillment—within its intended context of marriage between a man and woman—is one of the greatest blessings of God.

It's time we remove the shame from sex. God gave you sexual desires. Celebrate this gift—with your spouse. Remember, when God created everything else, he said, "It is good." When he created the two most sexual creatures on earth, he said, "It is *very good*."

Day 6
Inventory

When I was about ten, my dad gave my brother and me a summer job. For a few hours a week, we went to his office to count inventory. Dad owned his own company, where he worked as a sales rep. He sold electronics components from major factories to companies all over the country. He also stocked some parts at his office, to fill smaller orders.

These capacitors and reed relays were stored in small boxes. And they had to be counted from time to time. That's where Jim and I came in.

Dad paid us $1 for every box that we counted. But I made the most money. While Jim would count the boxes with dozens of tangled small parts, I'd open the boxes, and if there were a lot of parts inside, I'd close them back up. I only counted the boxes that had one or two parts.

That's how most of us do our personal inventory. We count empty boxes. When we look inside and find the complexity of tangled parts, we quickly shut the box and move on.

Paul said, "Examine yourselves" (2 Corinthians 13:5).

We all need to take an honest inventory of ourselves from time to time. Patrick Henry said it brilliantly: "Whatever anguish of spirit it may cost, I am willing to know the whole truth, to know the worst and to provide for it."

It is when you open the box and begin to untangle the worst parts that you find truth, freedom, and lasting recovery.

It's time to open the box and untangle the mixed-up parts.

Day 7
Bad Signs

I love funny signs. Let's consider a few examples.

In a London department store: "Bargain basement upstairs."

On the wall above the toilet in a public restroom: "This toilet out of order. Please use floor below."

Message on a leaflet: "If you cannot read this, please ask for assistance."

Message on a shop door: "We can repair anything. Knock on the door, as the bell does not work."

Those are bad signs. Let me suggest some other bad signs. You haven't been to a 12-Step meeting in two weeks. You have quit working the steps. You haven't called your sponsor in a while. You missed your morning devotions for the last three days.

The Bible says a lot about reading signs of things to come. Each time, we are told to respond to that sign. Jesus said, "When you see these things, recognize that he is near" (Matthew 24:33).

Signs point to a larger reality. If you see signs of slippage in your recovery, do something about it today.

What signs can others see that indicate you are serious about your recovery? Read the signs. Then respond accordingly.

Week 27
Scripture

"That Book, sir, is the Rock on which our Republic rests."

\- Andrew Jackson

THIS WEEK'S EXERCISE
Try the SOAP Method

Scripture reading and memorization must become a vital part of your recovery. I suggest you purchase a Life Recovery Bible. Our ministry actually gives these away for free. But regardless of which Bible you use, you need to be in the Word. That's why I send my Recovery Minute devotion to men and women from 15 countries around the world. That's why my second recovery book was a one-year devotional book for sex addicts. And that's why this workbook includes a devotional for every day of the year.

One of the great recovery stories in the Bible is the story of the paralytic, who suffered for 38 years. His account is recorded in John 5:1-15. For this week's exercise, read that passage, then take notes, based on the SOAP method.

S = Scripture
O = Observations
A = Application
P = Prayer

Here's how it works. Write down the **Scripture** verse that speaks to you most loudly, from this passage. Then jot down a few pertinent **Observations** from this passage. Third, write a few points of **Application** from the passage. Finally, write out a **Prayer**, based on this study.

Scripture: _____

Observations: _____

_____

_____

_____

_____

Application: _____

_____

_____

_____

_____

Prayer: _____

_____

_____

_____

_____

Day 1
Ferrari vs. Pinto

A leading voice on the porn effects on millennials is Alex Lerza, founder and CEO of The Recovery Tribe. Lerza summarizes the struggle of teens and young adults with the illustration of a car. He says of the emerging generation, "When it comes to sex and porn, they have a Ferrari engine, a Pinto set of brakes, and no owner's guide."

King David prayed, "Do not remember the sins of my youth and my rebellious ways" (Psalm 25:7).

As a young man, David struggled with the same temptations of today's generation. (And it's not just young men.) So what do we tell this new generation of young people—with a Ferrari engine, Pinto brakes, and no owner's guide? I suggest two things.

First, we tell them sex is not bad. Too often, in our effort to keep our kids on the "straight and narrow," we rely on shame. "All sex before marriage is sin," we tell them. Since they have not yet been married, what they hear us saying is, "All sex is sin." We tie sex to shame. That's bad.

Second, we give them the owner's guide. The good news is that we have an excellent owner's guide. We teach them biblical principles. We tell them that sex is beautiful, that they are beautiful, and that the God of sex created it for them—in the right time.

Cut out the secrets and lift the veil. The way to guide your kids down the right path is not to remove their engine or add anti-lock brakes, but to introduce them to the owner's guide.

Day 2
Lots-of-Stuff

There once lived a man in a far-away place that had so much stuff that they called it Stuffland. And this man had more stuff than anyone else. So they called him Lots-of-Stuff. He earned his stuff the old-fashioned way—through self-reliance and hard work. Then he heard about a new place with even more stuff. They called it New Stuffland. Lots-of-Stuff had to see it for himself, so he traveled to New Stuffland. And sure enough, he saw more stuff than he ever imagined.

Then a stranger approached, offering Lots-of-Stuff more stuff than he had ever imagined. But he could only have it on one condition. He had to give it away. And miraculously, the more stuff Lots-of-Stuff gave away, the more he got back.

The stranger in this parable is Jesus Christ. The "stuff" represents sobriety, and Lots-of-Stuff is you and me.

Recovery is not a reward for hard work and brilliance; it is a gift. But you cannot receive this gift until you meet the Giver—and commit to giving it away to others.

Jesus came to "seek and to save that which was lost" (Luke 19:10). He came for you and for me. He offers the gift of sobriety you could not earn on your own. The next step is yours.

You may have lots of stuff. You may even have lots of sobriety. But if you want the lasting gift of recovery, you must do two things—you must meet the Giver and share the gift with others.

Day 3
Fire in the Bones

President Reagan said of God's Word, "Within the covers of the Bible are the answers for all the problems men face."

When a skeptic expressed surprise at seeing him reading the Bible, Abraham Lincoln responded, "Take all that you can of this book upon reason, and the balance on faith, and you will live and die a happier man."

The prophet Jeremiah prayed, "Your word, O Lord, is like fire shut up in my bones" (20:9).

In recovery work, you will be encouraged to read from a lot of different sources. In 12-Step work, you will discover the white book, the green book, and the blue book. There are many online sources you can access. The number of books on recovery is limitless. And there is, of course, this daily devotion. (If you have to pick one, stick with my **Recovery Minute!**)

But often lost in the myriad assortment of helpful readings is this book we call the Bible. Let the same Book which inspired Presidents Lincoln and Reagan be your source of instruction and hope today.

In case you hadn't noticed, I have included Scripture in each of the 364 devotions in this book. Why? Because, as with Jeremiah, God's word is like a fire shut up in my bones.

May the fire of God's word warm your heart and guide your path today.

Day 4
Instructions

In recovery—and life—it is important to follow instructions. But it's not always easy, if these instructions don't make much sense. Here are a few examples of unclear instructions.

On a bag of Fritos: "You could be a winner! No purchase necessary. Details inside."

On a bar of Dial soap: "Directions: Use like regular soap."

On a kitchen knife: "Keep out of children."

On a string of Christmas lights: "For indoor or outdoor use only."

On a package of Sainsbury's Peanuts: "Warning—Contains nuts."

While recovery is not easy work, the instructions are pretty simple. They include such things as surrender, therapy, 12-Steps, and community. Where we get into trouble is not in trying to figure out what to do, but in doing what we have figured out.

The Bible says to "be doers of the word" (James 1:22). It's not that complicated. To find recovery, you must (a) read the instructions, then (b) do what they say.

You know the instructions. It's time to do what you know.

Day 5
Freedom's Key

"Then Jesus said to the Jews who had believed him, 'If you continue in my word, you really are my disciples. You will know the truth, and the truth will set you free'" (John 8:31-32). Jesus would later add that he was sent by God "to proclaim release to the captives, to set the oppressed free" (Luke 4:18). And he concluded his discourse in John with this promise: "If the Son sets you free, you really will be free" (8:36).

President Kennedy spoke of freedom when he said, "The great revolution in the history of man—past, present, and future—is the revolution of those determined to be free."

French philosopher Albert Camus added, "Freedom is nothing but a chance to be better."

That's all any of us want—a chance to be better. Freedom can give you that chance.

I have yet to meet the man who said, "I'm so glad I'm addicted to porn and sex." The good news is that there really is a way out.

Jesus is the key that open's freedom's door. Trust him today. Believe in him today. Rely on him today.

Do you want to get better? Do you want to be well? Then give your life to the Christ who promised "to set the captive free."

Day 6
Why Addicts Don't Get Well

I often tell friends that while some have the spiritual gift of preaching, encouragement, or leadership, my spiritual gift is worry. I'm good at it. *I'm really good at it!*

Worry's first cousin is fear. And that is our topic for today. It's the #1 reason many of us never get well. We struggle with fear. Specifically, we struggle with the fear of failure.

Whether you have been sober for one day or ten years, recovery presents daily challenges. There are times when you doubt yourself and your own recovery. There are times when you fall short of certain goals.

Why is fear such a problem in recovery? It's simple. Most addicts are perfectionists. They can't allow themselves to make mistakes or fall short—even a little bit. So they live in constant fear of failure.

The Partnership at Drugfree.org states that there are 23 million Americans living in successful recovery. But their study also went on to say that those not in recovery are eaten up with the fear of failure. And that's why addicts don't get well.

The Bible has the antidote for fear. "Perfect love casts out all fear" (1 John 4:18). Claim the love of God in your life, and you will take the first steps from fear to freedom.

Day 7
Better than Coffee

Since the early 1990s, Folgers has been the largest selling ground coffee in the United States. Many attribute the company's rise to the most famous coffee jingle of all time:

"The best part of wakin' up is Folgers in your cup."

We are a nation of coffee-drinkers. Every day, 64 percent of us drink at least one cup. Each day, more Americans drink coffee than pray (48 percent), read the Bible (14 percent), or exercise (five percent).

Do you drink too much coffee? The answer is probably yes if you meet any of the following criteria: (a) you play ping-pong by yourself, (b) you chew on other people's fingernails, or (c) you answer the door before the doorbell finishes ringing.

We love coffee because we love caffeine. And we love caffeine because we love stimulants. Kind of like porn—we think any boost of energy must be a good thing.

But every outside stimulant has a price to pay. The other day, a client told me his story: "My porn habit cost me my self-esteem and resulted in constant anxiety."

I'm not a coffee drinker. I never have been. So I don't know what kind of jolt that brings. But I do know what it is to drink in the Word of God every day. The old prophet said it like this: "Your words were found, and I ate them, and your words became to me a joy and the delight of my heart" (Jeremiah 15:16).

The effects of coffee—and porn—wear off. Drink in the Word of God today. I'm not saying you should quit drinking coffee; I'm just suggesting that a daily dose of God's Word is better.

Week 28
Ditches

"I'm one of those guys who has to have a constant
something going inside and in front of my face.
If not, I get in trouble."

- Garth Brooks

THIS WEEK'S EXERCISE
Define Your Ditch

In recovery, no matter how far you go down the road toward your goals, the ditch is still just as close on either side of the road. I have seen it happen far too often—a man with five, 10, or 15 years of sobriety falls to the temptations of illicit sexual activity.

It can happen so fast. An image, intrusive thought, memory, or some other trigger hits us in a weak moment, and we can fall. Let me be clear. *Any of us can fall—including you!* There are many ways to be ready and to stay sober. One important step is to recognize your weak spots. It is crucial to see the ditch on both sides of the road.

So here's the question of the day. If you fall, how will it happen? What are the two ditches that are the closest to your road today? And how do you plan to stay out of these two ditches?

Ditch #1: _____

How I plan to stay out of this ditch: _____
_____
_____

Ditch #2: _____

How I plan to stay out of this ditch: _____
_____
_____
_____

Day 1
Detours

Those who live in the north know just two seasons—winter and road repair. The harsh winter conditions bring ice and snow, which often buckle roads and create potholes. The result is that drivers in March and April are often faced with detours from their normal routes.

Some detours are the fault of the driver. A missed turn, lack of concentration, or refusal to ask for directions. They all mean rerouting our course. We take detours.

Barbara Bush said, "When you come to a roadblock, take a detour."

Zig Ziglar added, "Failure is a detour, not a dead-end street."

For many of us, our detour led us into a life of addiction. When we should have turned right, we went left. When we should have been in the Word, we were in the world.

But it's never too late to come back onto the main road. If you have driven off the intended path, there is an entrance ramp back to the thoroughfare of recovery. It's called "Jesus."

Jesus said, "I am the way" (John 14:6). Your habit has taken you off course. But it doesn't have to be a dead end. Follow Jesus back onto the road of sobriety and real recovery.

If you have drifted off course, it's not too late to get back on the main road. Follow Jesus. He is the only one who can take you where you want to be.

Day 2
A Great Fall

He was born in England in about 1870. He remains the most famous anthropomorphic egg of all time. Created by James William Elliott, he was popularized in America by actor George L. Fox. As a character and literary allusion, he has appeared in countless works of literature.

In 1954, a lyric was written in his honor, forever immortalizing his story:

Humpty Dumpty sat on a wall,
Humpty Dumpty had a great fall.
All the king's horses
And all the king's men

Couldn't put Humpty together again.

When a person lives a life of addiction, he is sitting on a wall. On one side is his public life; on the other, his hidden life. And he is fighting with everything he has to keep it all together. But eventually, every addict has a great fall. And with all his best effort and strength from within, he can't put himself together again.

In steps our Higher Power. The Bible says this about Christ: "By him all things consist" (Colossians 1:17).

Translation: After your great fall, Jesus can put you together again.

If you're sitting on the wall, you need to come down. But if you've already had a great fall, there's good news—Jesus can put you together again. But you've got to let Him.

Day 3
Why We Don't Get Well

When Jerald Maysworth decided to write a book on recovery, he knew what the first four words would be: "Everyone has an addiction." Paul said it like this: "All have sinned and fallen short" (Romans 3:23).

The fact that you are reading this indicates that you likely have an addiction or are close to someone who does. The next question is this: What are you going to do about it? As I see it, there are three reasons people don't get help with their addictions.

1. Denial. Brittany Meadows writes, "Addiction creates a form of smoke and mirrors that can make a person oblivious to the source or the root of their problems." A person will not seek help for a problem he does not first acknowledge.
2. Shame. While doubt can be a good thing, shame is always destructive. Doubt tells me, "You have done a bad thing." Shame says, "You are a bad person." When we live in shame, we are powerless to deal with life on life's terms.
3. Fear. Recovery is scary, hard, and long. It requires the addict to live in discomfort and to practice transparency. Recovery means being known. The process of healing can appear even more frightful than the addiction itself.

Have you fallen short? Of course, you have. We all have. But you are always within reach of the Savior and in line for recovery. But it will never happen as long as you choose to live in denial, shame, or fear.

You must go all in to find recovery. Denial, shame, and fear—these are your enemies. But they don't have to win.

Day 4
Pick One

Clay Olsen and his team at Fight the New Drug have done research on the question of why people turn to pornography. They have identified five reasons people look at porn.

1. For sexual arousal
2. For education about sex
3. Out of loneliness
4. Due to boredom
5. Response to peer pressure

Dr. Craig Cashwell, author of *Shadow of the Cross*, gives a deeper explanation. "We turn to porn in an effort to move toward or away from something."

What are you moving toward or away from?

The psalmist wrote, "Where shall I go from your Spirit? Or where shall I flee from your presence? If I ascend to heaven, you are there! If I make my bed in Sheol, you are there! If I take the wings of the morning and dwell in the uttermost parts of the sea, even there your hand shall lead me, and your right hand shall hold me" (Psalm 139:7-10).

You can't run to *porn* without running *from* God.

Draw a line in the sand. Porn or God? It's time to pick one.

Day 5
Direction

Recovery is not a destination, but a direction. It isn't something you achieve; it is something you pursue. You never get off the bus or complete the journey. You just keep going in the right direction.

When the prodigal son decided to leave home he really didn't have a destination in mind. "He got together all he had and set out for a distant country" (Luke 15:13). He didn't seem to have any particular country in mind; he simply headed out in a certain direction.

Notice what happened when the prodigal decided to return home. His father was back home, so the young man set out in that direction. But he never quite got there.

"While he was still a long way off, his father saw him and was filled with compassion for him; he ran to his son, threw his arms around him and kissed him" (15:20). Again, we see direction, not destination.

Theologian Rob Gronkowski said, "When you're growing up, you need to stay around people who are headed in the right direction and stay away from people who will take you in the wrong direction."

There it is again—direction. That is how we find recovery, one step at a time—in the right direction.

Don't be frustrated if you haven't gotten very far in your recovery. It's not about distance. It's not about destination. It's all about direction. So do all you really can do—take a few steps today—in the right direction.

Day 6
Enough Already

Do you ever feel like the task before you is greater than the strength within you? Meet Gideon.

While Gideon was doing his daily menial tasks, God showed up. One day he was threshing wheat; the next day he heard the voice of God: "Rescue Israel from the Midianites" (Judges 6:14).

Israel had lived in the shadow of the evil Midianite empire for years. Gideon pushed back at God's calling: "But Lord, how can I rescue Israel? My clan is the weakest in the whole tribe of Manasseh, and I am the least in my entire family!" (6:15).

Don't miss God's answer. Before Gideon had even stated his objection, God said, "Go with the strength you have" (6:14).

Did you catch that? *Go with the strength you have.* God didn't say, "Go with the strength you will have." Here's the point—God has already given you the strength you need to obey his will. If you are addicted to porn, you already have the strength you need to overcome. Your strength is in God—nothing else.

C.S. Lewis said, "He who has God and everything else has no more than he who has God only." I'm a big proponent of reading all the recovery material you can. But I love this, from Seneca, in *Letters from a Stoic*: "A multitude of books only gets in one's way."

So quit waiting for more knowledge or more strength to overcome. If you have God, you have all you need.

Day 7
No Longer Ashamed

On August 28, 1963, Martin Luther King, Jr., stood in front of the Lincoln Memorial and gave a speech. Perhaps you've heard of it. A small segment: "Free at last, free at last; thank God Almighty, I'm free at last."

I have a friend who is "free at last." T.C. Ryan was a highly successful pastor in Kansas City. Then his sex addiction became known, and his life was redirected—I would argue, into a better place. His book, *Ashamed No More*, offers hope for all of us who have walked similar paths. The premise of his book is that we can find freedom in Christ and live the rest of our lives beyond shame.

A little-known prophet by the name of Zephaniah addressed this subject. Speaking of a future deliverance of God's children, he said, "On that day you will no longer need to be ashamed" (3:11).

When you seek God in Christ Jesus, and when you go all in with recovery, shame has no place in your life. God has set you free, so live like it!

Have you embraced a life of recovery and integrity? Then say it with me: "Free at last, free at last; thank God Almighty, I'm free at last."

Week 29
Choices

"Life is a matter of choices, and every
choice you make makes you."

- John Maxwell

THIS WEEK'S EXERCISE
Eat Some Starburst

You make your choices, then your choices make you. Decisions of your past—both good and bad—have become a part of your DNA. You can't go back. While you do get to write a whole new ending to your life, you cannot write a new beginning. One of the things we must learn in order to go forward is to quit trying to have a better past.

In recovery, we acknowledge our past and try to move on. But the abuse still happened. The trauma left enduring scars. The isolation shaped who we became. And then we, as addicts, fell into patterns that damaged us and those closest to us. But in recovery, we realize that God can use us this way, in ways he could not have used us otherwise.

This will be the tastiest exercise of the year. Buy a pack of Starburst candy. Then remove two of the individually wrapped candies. They must be of different flavors. Now, put these two together, and begin mashing them and twisting them until they become one. Keep working with the new product until the two colors are intertwined as one. This will take several minutes.

Once the two have become one, eat the new Starburst that is in your hand.
Now, answer the following questions.

1. Which two flavors did you start out with? _____ and _____

2. Once you meshed them into one, could you have separated them back into the two individual pieces that you started with? Why or why not? _____
_____

3. Did the new product taste like either of the first two? _____

4. One candy represents you as a person. The other represents a choice you have made to act out in the past. In what ways did this choice change you permanently? _____ _____

_____

5. Do you think good choices change who you become, as well? _____

Day 1
Truth & Consequences

On his last day in office, Governor Bill Richardson of New Mexico did what every other governor had done for the past 130 years. He refused to issue an official pardon for notorious outlaw Billy the Kid.

Also known as Henry McCarty, "The Kid" was responsible for at least 20 deaths. But in 1879, New Mexico Governor Lew Wallace promised him a pardon in exchange for his testimony against three men accused of killing a one-armed lawyer during the Lincoln County Wars. But Wallace reneged on his promise, and Billy the Kid escaped from prison, killing four guards. He was eventually tracked down and killed on July 14, 1881.

To this day, there are those who still call for Billy's pardon. But that pardon has not come, and probably never will.

Here's the deal—choices have consequences.

The old prophet said, "The soul that sins will surely die" (Ezekiel 18:4). Addiction will take you further than you want to go, keep you longer than you want to stay, and cost you more than you want to pay.

You don't need to apologize for an addiction. But what you do about it is on you.

Day 2
Brave Heart

In the closing scene of *Braveheart*, William Wallace was being tortured and executed for leading a rebellion against the evil English king. Even at the moment of his greatest pain, he still longed for his countrymen to experience something he was giving his life for—freedom.

With freedom comes tension. The apostle wrote, "For you have been called to live in freedom, my brothers and sisters. But don't use your freedom to satisfy your sinful nature. Instead, use your freedom to serve one another" (Galatians 5:13).

Let's talk about it. Thucydides said, "The secret to happiness is freedom, and the secret to freedom is courage."

Indeed, it takes courage to use freedom wisely.

You are free to make bad decisions. You are free to satisfy your sinful nature whenever and however you want. But anyone can do that. You are better than that.

Do what you know is right. Have the courage to do what *is* right instead of what *feels* right.

God has set you free through faith in Christ. You can now go in one of two directions. You can use your freedom to satisfy your sinful nature, or you can use your freedom to serve others. One road is easy. The other is paved with courage. The next move is yours.

Day 3
Banquet of Consequences

We hear it all the time. "Life isn't fair." But is that really true?

It's not fair that you were emotionally abandoned by your parents. Abuse isn't fair. Neglect, family history, maltreatment—none of them are fair.

The American Psychiatric Association states that three million children experience abuse in America each year. The World Health Organization says this abuse comes in four forms: physical, sexual, emotional, and psychological. It's all abuse, and none of it is fair.

But at some point, we are responsible for our own decisions. What happens to us is not our fault. But our destructive responses are.

The prophet said, "The day of the Lord is near for all nations. As you have done, it will be done to you; your deeds will return upon your own head" (Obadiah 15).

Robert Louis Stevenson said, "Sooner or later, everyone sits down to a banquet of consequences."

Your choices bring a banquet of consequences. You can blame your past or you can change your future. Those are your two options.

Day 4
Healing

Popeye said to Bluto, "Even though you're bigger than me, you can't win, 'cause you're bad, and the good always wins over the bad."

The truth is that good *can* win over the bad, those suffering from addictions *can* get well, and healing *can* take place. Helen Keller was right: "Although the world is full of suffering, it is also full of the overcoming of it."

Healing can come—to your life and to your marriage. Jeremiah prayed, "Heal me, O Lord, and I will be healed; save me and I will be saved, for you are the one I praise" (17:14).

Addiction literature asserts that healing comes spiritually, emotionally, and physically. But, as Carl Townsend said, "All healing is first a healing of the heart."

How does this work, exactly? Carol Alexander, Director of the Graduate School at Trinity Bible College in North Dakota, writes, "You can confront your hurtful moments, deal with the pain, and move on. The first decision you have to make is to confront the memory, and that can hurt. But it is the first and necessary step in the journey to healing."

The good can win over the bad. Healing can win over the addiction. But healing is a *choice*, not a *chance*. And it begins in the heart, when you surrender your life and your will over to God.

Day 5
Decisions, Decisions

A reporter writing a story on Florida's citrus industry entered a shed where a worker was sorting oranges. As the oranges tumbled down a conveyer belt, the man put large oranges into large holes, small oranges into small holes, and bruised oranges into another hole.

The worker performed his boring task perfectly, when the reporter stepped in. "How can you stand doing this all day—putting oranges in the holes?"

The man replied, "You don't know the half of it! From the time I get here until the time I leave, it's decisions, decisions, decisions."

Life is all about decisions.

Chuck Swindoll says, "The difference in your life tomorrow will be the decisions you make today."

C.S. Lewis observed, "Every time you make a choice you are turning the central part of either into a heavenly creature or into a hellish creature."

In recovery, we talk a lot about process, boundaries, brain chemistry, community, accountability, and more. But every time you are tempted—and you will be—it boils down to a decision.

We have this promise. "If you wander off the road to the right or the left, you will hear his voice behind you saying, 'Here is the road. Follow it'" (Isaiah 30:21).

Day 6
Relativity

"When you are courting a nice girl, an hour seems like a second. When you sit on a red-hot cinder, a second seems like an hour. That's relativity" (Albert Einstein).

Relativity transcends God's universe. From courting a nice girl to sitting on a red-hot cinder to sex addiction, relativity is at play.

Let me explain. When living in the depths of any addiction, a second is a lifetime. The pain lingers, the memories haunt, and the shame is absolutely unrelenting. But every day in recovery is like a good movie. When it's over, we only want more.

Sexually compulsive behaviors have their root in trauma, isolation, and abuse. But each action, taken outside the bounds of God's law, is sin. And like sitting on the red-hot cinder, each sin has consequences.

Isaiah said, "But your iniquities have made a separation between you and your God, and your sins have hidden his face from you so that he does not hear" (59:2).

The good news is that, at the very second we are caving to our lust, God is at work. The pain of his correction is necessary and good. Charles Stanley said, "Regardless of the source, adversity is always a powerful tool in the Lord's hands." And John Piper adds, "If we are on the right track, the only hope for seeing the glory of God is that he cut away the diamond-hard, idolatrous substitutes for the glory of God that are packed into the template of our hearts."

Day 7
Royal Gorge

Several years ago, while sponsoring our church's high school camp, I rafted the Arkansas River through the famed Royal Gorge near Colorado Springs. I had rafted dozens of times, so the threat of Class 5 rapids held no fear. I joined a group of high school athletes in the raft, and off we went, floating gently downstream.

But in a couple of hours, the pace quickly increased. And just ahead was the most terrifying waterfall imaginable. I wanted out, but it was too late. We went over the falls sideways, and we found ourselves lodged against a rock. Water was pouring into the raft. It took several minutes and all of our collective strength to break free.

In the Sexaholics Anonymous "white book," we read about "The Problem." It reads, "Like revelers riding a raft down the river of pleasure, we were unaware of the awesome power of the rapids or the whirlpool ahead."

Millions of men have set their boat into the gentle waters of "soft porn," dating apps, or singles bars. No problem—at first. But the gentle current became Class 5 rapids, and there was no way out. Surviving the deadly falls became the only option.

The good news is that you have a choice. No one is forcing you into the boat. If you're already in the raft, pull aside before the gentle stream becomes a deadly fall from which there is no escape.

Week 30
Accountability

"People do what you inspect, not what you expect."

- Louis V. Gerstner, Jr.

THIS WEEK'S EXERCISE
Get an Accountability Partner

I like to say it a lot—God will only heal what we reveal. There are two extremes to which I see recovering addicts run. They either (a) tell too many people their story, or they (b) tell their story to no one. Let's focus on that second extreme.

Many of us have cried out, "All I need is God!" And that sounds really good. The problem is that the God we need wired us for fellowship. More than that, we are wired for accountability. That's why the Bible promises healing when we confess our struggles to another human being.

There is usually that "one" magazine, website, computer file, TV show, or person. Because you tried to find victory on your own—and failed—you must now become accountable to one other human being.

You need an accountability partner. This is a person with whom you will meet regularly (weekly, if possible). You will tell him or her your struggles, slips, and temptations. You will give him or her permission to ask the tough questions about your daily sobriety. It will be best if this person meets the following criteria:

He or she is the same sex as you.
He or she is in recovery themselves.
He or she can be trusted.
He or she will pray for you.
He or she offers godly wisdom.
He or she is a committed Christ-follower.
He or she will ask you the hard questions.

For this exercise, you need to do three things: (a) decide whom you will ask to be your accountability partner, (b) decide when you will ask him or her, and (c) actually ask him or her. Let's start with the first two parts of this assignment.

Who you will ask: _____

When you will ask him or her: _____

Day 1
Lucy and Ethel

In life—and recovery—we need friends. Perhaps no television show ever depicted a strong friendship quite like the one between Lucy and Ethel on *I Love Lucy*. In one episode, we discover the essence of friendship.

Ethel: "You always drag me into your crazy schemes!"

Lucy: "Well, this is one time I can do it without you."

Ethel: "What's wrong with me all of a sudden?"

Lucy: "Well, alright, Ethel, you can come along if you want to."

Ethel: "No, I don't want to. I just wanted you to ask me."

King David had an unusually close bond with his friend Jonathan. So close was their relationship that the Scriptures tell us that at Jonathan's funeral, David lamented, "I am distressed for you, my brother Jonathan" (2 Samuel 1:26).

Ethel didn't need to be with Lucy all the time. She just needed to be asked. Who have you asked to do life with? You cannot win the victory over temptation, addiction, and isolation alone. As David needed Jonathan and Lucy needed Ethel, you need someone in your life—for encouragement, strength, and accountability.

Day 2
Safety Net

Andy Stanley says the greatest question ever is: *What is the wise thing to do?* But the answer is not always clear. This leads to what Andy calls the second greatest question ever: *What do you think is the wise thing to do?*

Solomon said it like this: "Plans go wrong for lack of advice; many advisers bring success" (Proverbs 15:22). He also wrote, "There is safety in having many advisers" (Proverbs 11:14).

It's what I call the safety net. In recovery, none of us is as strong as all of us. Michael Leahy, founder of Bravehearts, says that only one man in 10,000 gets well on his own. We need each other.

To find successful recovery, you will need several people in your corner: a therapist, a pastor or priest, a sponsor, sponsees, 12-Step friends, and more.

When I am struggling, I call my pastor. Sometimes I call a mentor in the field of sex addiction. Other times, I call my sponsor.

The important thing is not *who* you call, but *that* you call. Can you surround yourself with helpful advisers and still slip or relapse? Absolutely! But if you go it alone, I can almost guarantee you will have a relapse. You need many advisers. That is about the best safety net you will ever find.

Day 3
One Is the Loneliest Number

Those great theologians, Three Dog Night, sang, "One is the loneliest number." And they were right.

Solomon wrote, "Two are better than one, because they have a good return for their labor; if either of them falls down, the other can help them up" (Ecclesiastes 4:9-10).

You will never go far in life—especially in recovery—on your own. You need someone to whom you can be accountable.

A little-known football player named Tom Brady knows a little about teamwork. He said of his coach, "Coach Belichick holds us accountable every day. We appreciate when he's tough on us. He gets the best out of us."

And basketball coach Lenny Wilkins said, "The most important quality I look for in a player is accountability."

In *Five Values for the Workplace*, Robert Dilenschneider identified the following keys to success on any team: integrity, accountability, diligence, perseverance, and discipline.

There's that word again—*accountability*. Successful recovery cannot be achieved alone. You need a sponsor, a counselor, and a group. You need accountability—because in recovery one is the loneliest number.

Day 4
Fully Accountable

One of the great examples of an accountability relationship is found in the Bible. It involved two unlikely friends, David and Jonathan, whom we introduced a couple of days ago. Theirs was an unlikely relationship because it was Jonathan's father who tried to have David killed—repeatedly.

This is their story: "After David had finished talking with Saul, Jonathan became one in spirit with David . . . and Jonathan made a covenant with David" (1 Samuel 18:1, 3).

David accomplished amazing things as long as he maintained accountability in his life. And the same can be true for you. What makes accountability work? I suggest five things.

1. Accountability will accelerate your progress.
2. Accountability provides a clear measure of your work.
3. Accountability will keep you engaged and on track.
4. Accountability will hold you responsible.
5. Accountability will validate your direction.

Nothing great can be done by isolation. And there is nothing greater that you will ever achieve than lasting recovery. So connect with your sponsor or someone else in recovery and become accountable to them. That will provide your best chance of success.

Find one person to whom you can be accountable. This may be your 12-Step sponsor, a member of a men's or ladies' group. Then initiate contact with this person and prayerfully pursue a relationship of accountability.

Day 5
Shakespearean Wisdom

Let's begin our day with a little Shakespeare: "This above all: to thine own self be true, and it must follow, as the night the day, thou canst not then be false to any man" (*Hamlet*).

Translation: You need others in your life, but any relationship must be rooted in total honesty.

In recovery, pick your friends carefully. You need a sponsor—someone who has been where you are and is now where you're going. Solomon's oft-quoted words still ring true: "As iron sharpens iron, one man sharpens another" (Proverbs 27:17).

You need people in your life who play two positions on your team: (a) honesty, and (b) encouragement.

I like the way Bernard M. Baruch said it. "Be who you are and say what you feel, because those who mind don't matter and those who matter don't mind."

You need people in your life who matter, people whose love is unconditional. You must be true to yourself, then honest with your sponsor and others. Open the door to those who share their wisdom with a mind that is honest and a heart that encourages.

You need others in your life, to lead and encourage your recovery. These relationships must be rooted in honesty. But first, you must be honest with yourself.

Day 6
A King Gone Bad

Jeroboam came from good stock. His dad (Solomon) was king, and his grandfather (David) was king. Now the mantle fell on his shoulders. But Jeroboam did not wear that mantle well.

The young leader suffered from two major character flaws:

1. He persisted in wrong behaviors.
2. He failed to build any relationships of accountability.

Jeroboam persisted in a life of apostasy. He ignored God's laws about priesthood (Numbers 3:10) by appointing unqualified priests. God brought a prophet into his life whose name is not given. Eighteen times throughout 1 Kings 13, he is simply identified as "the man of God." This prophet warned Jeroboam to change his ways. But when he persisted in disobedience, "this became a great sin and resulted in the utter destruction of Jeroboam's dynasty from the face of the earth" (1 Kings 13:34).

Persistence in the wrong direction plus no accountability—this is a formula for disaster. So what about you? Are you hanging onto unhealthy behaviors? Do you lack real accountability in your life? The good news is that both of these dangerous choices can be erased in a day.

You need to change your old behaviors, while inserting accountability into your life—starting today.

Day 7
The Kind of Friends You Need

Robin Dunbar, a British anthropologist, has conducted a study of how many friends the average person has. He concludes that we are generally connected, on average, to 148 people. Dr. Marie Hartwell-Walker has delved deeper into this study and concluded that of these 148, about 15 can be considered actual friends.

A Gallup Poll finds that the average American claims to have nine "close friends," but the poll is not clear as to what "close" means.

Friends are an important component of recovery.

Jesus valued friendships, as "he lay down his life for his friends" (John 15:13). Solomon believed in friends so strongly that he laid out specific requirements for finding the right friends (Proverbs 22:24-25).

So what kind of friends do you need? Ralph Waldo Emerson said it like this: "It is one of the blessings of old friends that you can afford to be stupid with them."

How many friends know about your "stupidity"? You need to be held accountable for any future acts of stupidity that you might commit. And that is where friends come in.

You cannot find recovery on your own. So ask God to lead you to the right friends that can walk this journey with you.

Week 31
Desperation

"We must act boldly because the situation
is so desperate."

- Romeo and Juliet
Act 4, Scene 1

THIS WEEK'S EXERCISE
What Are You Willing to Do?

Until you get desperate, you won't get well. I have yet to meet the person who achieved lasting sobriety casually. You can't sprinkle a little recovery work into your normal lifestyle and expect to get well. When I assess a new client, I can usually tell within a few minutes whether he will find success or not. It's all a matter of desperation. I see various levels on the desperation scale:

- "I may have a problem."
- "I have a problem."
- "This is an addiction."
- "I would like to get well."
- "I need help to get well."
- "I will work to get well."
- "I will be sick if I don't get well."
- "I'll die if I don't get well."

It is when we "hit bottom" that we get well. Why is this? Because we have to become desperate. Finding sexual sobriety is the hardest thing most of us will ever do. For some, it requires attending 90 recovery meetings in 90 days. For most, it requires therapy. For all, it requires honesty and hard work.

If you are 90% in, you are 100% out!

What you do to find recovery is critical. But what matters even more is that which you are *willing to do*.

Here's a list. Check the things you are willing to do to get well, if they prove to be key components to your recovery plan.

_____ Do therapy

_____ Join a 12-Step group

_____ Complete this workbook

_____ See a C.S.A.T.

_____ Sell something to pay for therapy

_____ Work the 12 Steps

_____ Do a full clinical disclosure

_____ Take a polygraph

_____ Work with a sponsor

_____ Become a sponsor

_____ Get on Covenant Eyes

_____ Go to an inhouse treatment center

_____ Attend 90 meetings in 90 days

_____ Do nightly check-ins with your spouse

Day 1
Desperation

Hippocrates said, "Desperate times call for desperate measures." The man seemed to understand addiction. Desperation is the birthplace of recovery. You will never find lasting, sustainable recovery without it. You have to want recovery more than anything else.

I can't think of a more desperate situation in the Bible than that of Lazarus. The man was dying, so his sisters came to Jesus and pled for him to heal their brother. Jesus responded, "This sickness will not end in death" (John 11:4). And then, two days later, Lazarus died.

So what gives?

Notice what Jesus *did not say*. He didn't say Lazarus wouldn't die. He said the sickness would not *end in death*.

Think about it. If Jesus had healed Lazarus before he died, he would have just been another nameless guy in the Bible. What made Lazarus famous was not his healing, but his resurrection.

God is the master of the resurrection. Think about your own recovery. Your addiction may have killed your marriage, your job, your finances, and your self-esteem. But God's promise is that it won't end there. God always gets the final word.

Addiction brings death. But in death we find resurrection and recovery. When we rely fully on him, we discover that, as with Lazarus, "this sickness will not end in death."

Day 2
Did Jesus Really Say That?

Jesus came upon a man who had been sick for 38 years. We can assume the man had tried everything: doctors, religion, and home remedies. Still he was sick. He had played his last card. He was out of options. So he looked to Jesus.

And Jesus asked him the strangest question: "Do you want to be well?" (John 5:6). Was that a serious question? Sure, he wanted to be well! Who wouldn't?

But Jesus' question really wasn't one of desire, but desperation. "Do you *really* want to be well?" He told the man—who could not walk—to pick up his mat and walk. That required a willingness to look the part of a fool. What if the healing didn't really take place?

But when he did the improbable, Jesus did the impossible. And the man was healed.

The first key to freedom is desperation. Most of us are more comfortable with old problems than new solutions. So we never find freedom.

Real freedom comes when we are more desperate for God than we are for his blessings.

St. Augustine said, "To fall in love with God is the greatest romance; to seek him the greatest adventure; to find him, the greatest human achievement."

Perhaps you have been mired in years of pain and struggle. The answer is found in this question. Do you want to get well? *Really?*

Day 3
Bottoms Up

Every person I've seen get well had one thing in common. They hit bottom.

The Old Testament tells the story of such a woman. When a new widow was out of food and had become desperate, she cried out to Elisha for help. Without her husband to provide for her, the widow feared she would lose her sons to slavery. She needed to provide for them immediately, but she had precious few resources, and her family was hungry. Elisha asked her what she had in the house.

The widow had only a little oil. "She went and told the man of God, and he said, 'Go, sell the oil and pay your debts. You and your sons can live on what is left'" (2 Kings 4:7). In obedience, she started to fill the jars with oil, and God miraculously multiplied the oil.

The woman shifted her focus from what she had *lost* to what she had *left*. And then the blessings began to flow.

F.B. Meyer said, "We must get to the end of ourselves before God can begin in us." Teddy Roosevelt said it like this: "When you reach the end of your rope, tie a knot and hang on."

Perhaps you've come to the end of your rope. That's a good place to be. That means you have hit bottom. You have nowhere else to turn but to the God you should have turned to all along.

If you are to the end of your rope, if you are truly desperate, you are in a good place. Why? Because it is only when you let go that God takes over.

Day 4
The Sinking Feeling

That sinking feeling.

Peter knew it well. In an instant, he went from hero to goat, from walking on water to nearly drowning.

"Peter got down out of the boat, walked on water and came toward Jesus. But when he saw the wind, he was afraid and, beginning to sink, cried out, 'Lord, save me!' Immediately Jesus reached out his hand and caught him" (Matthew 14:29-31).

Like Peter, many of us walked on top of it all. But our addictions caught up to us. We began to sink. But Jesus majors in catching those who sink.

In 1912, in Saugatuck, Connecticut, James Rowe read this passage about Peter, then jotted down a few words on paper, writing from his personal experience as the impoverished son of a copper miner.

I was sinking deep in sin, far from the peaceful shore,
Very deeply stained within, sinking to rise no more;
But the Master of the sea heard my despairing cry,
From the waters lifted me, now safe am I.
Love lifted me, love lifted me!
When nothing else could help, love lifted me!

Do you know that sinking feeling? Turn to Christ. He majors in rescuing those who are sinking deep in sin, far from the peaceful shore.

Day 5
39 Failures

Miriam Hargrave, of Wakefield, England, holds a dubious record for perseverance. After 31 attempts at passing her driving test, she told a newspaper, "I've spent all my savings and my husband has threatened to leave me if I don't give up trying."

But at the age of 62, Miriam finally realized her dream. On August 3, 1970, she passed the test—on her 40th attempt. (Unfortunately, Miriam had spent $720 on 212 lessons, leaving her no money with which to purchase a car.)

Paul told the church at Rome, "Never be lacking in zeal" (Romans 12:11).

I can't think of a single activity that requires more zeal than recovery. We have to be all in. The man who is 90 percent committed will ultimately end up in the same place as the man who is just 10 percent committed.

My old pastor, Dr. Cecil Sewell, likes to say, "If Jesus isn't Lord *of all*, he isn't Lord *at all*." That all-or-nothing mentality works in recovery, as well.

Maybe you're like Miriam. You have failed the test 39 times. That just means you are that much closer to your goal.

Remain zealous. Never lose your passion to be well.

Day 6
The Desperation Cycle

Buried deep in the historic writings of the Old Testament is the story of King Jehoahaz. His reign over Israel lasted for 17 years. In his early years, the king "did what was evil in the Lord's sight" (2 Kings 13:2). His rebellion against God resulted in judgment, as the army of Aram defeated Israel on multiple battlefields. "Then Jehoahaz prayed for the Lord's help, and the Lord heard his prayer" (13:4). Now, "Israel lived in safety again as they had in former days" (13:5).

Then the people did what so many do. When times were good once again, they returned to their old ways. "They continued to sin, and the king of Aram trampled them like dust under his feet" (13:6-7).

King Jehoahaz is a case study on addiction. Notice the cycle: (a) wrong actions, (b) price to pay, (c) remorse and repentance, (d) God's restoration, (e) return to the old ways.

I see it all the time. In recovery literature, it's what we call "half measures." They avail us nothing.

Jim Carrey nailed it. "I don't think human beings learn anything without desperation. Desperation is a necessary ingredient to learning anything."

Where are you in the desperation cycle? It's time to get off the crazy train. When God forgives and restores, you can follow the example of Jehoahaz and return to your own ways. But you don't have to.

243

Day 7
The Beginning of Success

Until you get desperate you won't get well. Tony Robbins said it well: "Success begins with desperation."

Jesus once dealt with a woman who was truly desperate.

"A Gentile woman who lived there came to him, pleading, 'Have mercy on me, O Lord, Son of David! For my daughter is possessed by a demon that torments her severely.' Jesus said to the woman, 'I was sent only to help God's lost sheep—the people of Israel.' But she came and worshiped him, pleading again, 'Lord, help me!' Jesus responded, 'It isn't right to take food from the children and throw it to the dogs.' She replied, 'That's true, Lord, but even dogs are allowed to eat the scraps that fall beneath their master's table.' 'Dear woman,' Jesus said to her, 'your faith is great. Your request is granted.' And her daughter was instantly healed" (Matthew 15:22-28).

Are you that desperate for God's movement in your life? Are you willing to pray as though your recovery depends upon God, and then work as though it all depends upon you?

Until you get desperate you won't get well.

Week 32
Giving Back

"My own experience about all the blessings I've had in my life is that the more I give away, the more that comes back."

\- Ken Blanchard

THIS WEEK'S EXERCISE
Become a Sponsor

Helping others can be a vital part of your personal recovery from sexual addiction. This is what Step 12 is all about. As of this writing, I am sponsoring men (apart from this ministry) in five states. I always tell them, "I'm doing this for me." The fact is, when we help others, we help ourselves.

I hear something important in every 12-Step meeting. I pray the same will be true with the groups our ministry leads. But I also learn and grow by sponsoring other men. Dr. Doug Weiss writes, "Helping another struggling sex addict will strengthen your faith and remind you of the precious gift you have been given in your recovery."

The more you help others, the more you will be helped. You need to find ways to give back, to help others in their recovery. You can start by sponsoring someone else in their recovery work.

Pray and ask God to lay someone on your heart who needs your help. Then set a time to visit with them and make yourself available to lead them through their recovery process.

Date I prayed for God to lead me to someone in need: _____

Names of three men I might help or sponsor:

    1. _____

    2. _____

    3. _____

Date I will talk to one of these men: _____

Day 1
Father Damien

Tourists visit the Hawaiian Island of Molokai to enjoy the beaches and charm. But Father Damien came for a different reason. He came to help people die. You see, lepers came here first, starting in about 1840. They lived in isolation, on a tract of land set aside just for them.

When Father Damien heard of their plight, he begged with his supervisors to let him move to Molokai, to live with the lepers. The year was 1873. Damien said, "I want to sacrifice myself for the lepers."

Damien entered the world of the lepers. He dressed their sores, hugged their children, and buried their dead. Eventually, he would contract their disease. On April 15, 1889, Father Damien died of leprosy.

Father Damien did for the Molokai lepers what Jesus did for each of us. Not content to simply "treat" man, Jesus became a man. He joined the human race. The Bible says, "It was necessary for him to be made in every respect like us so that he could be our merciful and faithful High Priest before God" (Hebrews 2:17).

You can overcome every temptation because of what Jesus has done. Not content to look down on us from above, He has joined us. You are not alone. Because he became man, Christ knows exactly what you are going through, and he will walk with you every step of the way.

Recognize that you are not alone. Embrace the One who understands every temptation you will ever face—because he's been there. In fact, he still is.

Day 2
It's Why We Are Here

W.H. Auden said, "We are all here on earth to help others. Why they are here, I have no idea."

Auden is actually on to something. We are here for others, not ourselves. Les Brown said it like this: "Help others achieve their dreams and you will achieve yours." That is especially true in recovery.

Charles Plumb was an American pilot in the Vietnam War. When his plane was shot down, he ejected and parachuted into the jungle, where the Viet Cong captured him and held him captive for six years. Years later, Plumb was dining at a restaurant with his wife when a stranger approached him. He said, "You are Charles Plumb, aren't you? You were shot down over Vietnam."

Plumb asked the stranger who he was. "I'm the man who packed your parachute that day. I guess it worked!"

Plumb gives speeches across America. He tells that story, then asks his audiences, "Who packed your parachute?"

Recovery is a team sport. We find recovery by helping others find recovery. One of the best things you can do to secure your own recovery is to help someone else secure theirs.

The Bible says, "There will never cease to be poor in the land. Therefore, I command you, 'You shall open wide your hand to your brother, to the needy and to the poor in your land'" (Deuteronomy 15:11).

Day 3
12th Step

Recovery is not complete until we work the 12th Step: "Having had a spiritual awakening as the result of these steps, we tried to carry the message to others." Recovery is not just about what God is doing *in* us; it's about what God is doing *through* us.

Poet Ella Wheelcox said it like this: "There are only two kinds of people on earth today, two kinds of people, no more, I say; not the good and the bad, for 'tis well understood, that the good are half bad and the bad are half good. No, the two kinds of people on earth I mean are the people who lift and the people who lean."

It's never too soon to practice the 12th Step. From day one, you need to start giving back. When you go to your next 12-Step meeting, find the newcomer and give him your number. Help set up the room. Look for the person who doesn't seem to fit in and become his friend. Find the man with no sobriety and praise him for just showing up.

One day, Jesus bragged on a woman who gave very little, but who gave it all. Comparing her to bigger givers, he said, "They all gave out of their wealth; but she, out of her poverty, put in everything—all she had to live on" (Mark 12:44).

Martin Luther King, Jr., wrote, "Somewhere along the way, we must learn that there is nothing greater than to do something for others."

Learn to give back. Find someone who needs a word of encouragement, and give it to them. And by being the healer, you will be healed.

Day 4
The Great Conductor

Born in Budapest in 1897, George Szell was one of the most gifted pianists in the world. But no one remembers George Szell the pianist. They remember George Szell the conductor.

By age 20, Szell was conducting the Strasbourg Opera. By 27, he led the Berlin State Opera, and by 35, he had migrated to the United States and become lead conductor at the Metropolitan Opera House in New York City. For 25 years, Szell was recognized as the world's greatest conductor.

What was the key to Szell's success? One thing, he said. "Early in life, I decided to not focus on being the best pianist, but to help others be the best."

That is the definition of leadership—helping others. James defined religion as "visiting orphans and widows in their affliction, and to keep oneself unstained from the world" (James 1:27).

In recovery, we can only go so far if we don't pour our lives into others. The most sober people I know are the ones who do the most to sponsor newcomers, make calls, and give back. As we say in every 12-Step meeting, "The measure we gave was the measure we got back."

Look beyond yourself. Find someone this week who needs you and give them your time and your wisdom. You will discover that the best way to secure your own sobriety is by helping others secure theirs.

Day 5
Fit to Be Used

In *Authentic Christianity*, Ray Stedman writes, "There is nothing so exciting as being an instrument in the hand of God, or realizing that we are fit to be used."

David faced this challenge long before he became king. He had one gift. He was really good with a slingshot. When David was a teenager out in the shepherds' fields, he had spent hours practicing while he was caring for his father's sheep. He could have thought, "God, why didn't you give me an impressive gift? Why did you give me just one talent? I'm an expert with a slingshot. Big deal! That's never going to take me anywhere!"

There once lived a man who came to wish that David had embraced that negative attitude, and that David had given up on his gift. That man's name was Goliath.

The Bible says, "God chose what is foolish in the world to shame the wise; God chose what is weak in the world to shame the strong" (1 Corinthians 1:27).

You may have just one gift. Join the ranks of Leonardo Da Vinci, Ludwig van Beethoven, Christopher Columbus, William Shakespeare, Muhammad Ali, and Michael Jordan. One trick ponies—all of them! And I'm sure they all heard it growing up. "You'll never amount to anything by painting, composing, exploring, writing, fighting, or shooting a basketball!"

What does this have to do with recovery? Everything! Part of recovery is helping others. You need to do what a boy named David did. Unwrap your gift, whether it is a slingshot or something else. Then start using your gift to help others. In the process, you will help yourself.

Day 6
How to Help Yourself

The AA "Big Book" offers a detailed description of the 12th Step. A quote from this passage: "Even the newest of newcomers finds undreamed rewards as he tries to help his brother alcoholic, the one who is even blinder than he" (p. 109).

For each of us in recovery, there is someone out there who is "blinder."

The final piece to the puzzle—which sadly, too few discover—is the 12th Step. It is here that we go all in to help others. In the process, they help us.

Elbert Hubbard wrote, "Down in their hearts, wise men know the truth: the only way to help yourself is to help others."

One of the exciting things about helping others is that you never know who you're helping, and what they can become in their own recovery.

One day, Moses sent Joshua off to lead the troops into battle against the Amalekites. Moses would stay back, holding his hands up with his staff in his hands, symbolic of God's power to bring victory to his children. But Moses' hands became weary. "When Moses' hands grew tired, Aaron and Hur held his hands up—one on each side—so that his hands remained steady until sunset" (Exodus 17:12). And the Israelites were victorious.

Day 7
It's Why You Are Here

I'm writing today out of my personal devotional experience. In my daily readings from the Life Recovery Bible, I came across this verse the other day. This wasn't the first time I've found this verse, but it might be the first time this verse found me.

"Through him [Christ] God created everything in the heavenly realm and on earth. He made the things we can see and the things we cannot see—such as thrones, kingdoms, rulers, and authorities in the unseen world. Everything was created through him and for him" (Colossians 1:16).

Catch that last part—*"Everything was created through him and for him."*

Everything was created for him. I'm part of "everything". So are you. And that makes us special. Imagine that! The God of the universe created you for His pleasure. That's your purpose in life—to please Him.

When you are faced with your next temptation, keep this in mind. That decision affords you an incredible opportunity. In that moment, you can put a smile on the face of God—if you make the right choice.

Your body was created for God. Your mind was created for Him. Your talents, intelligence, your personality—they were all created for God. Let that sink in. Then live this day in a way that fulfills Colossians 1:16.

Week 33
Prayer

"Prayer does not change God, but it does change the person who prays."
- Soren Kierkegaard

THIS WEEK'S EXERCISE
Pray According to A.C.T.S.

The disciples of Jesus did not ask him how to pray. They pled, "Teach us to pray" (Luke 11:1). And then Jesus gave them what has become known as The Lord's Prayer. The point is not so much *how* we pray, but *that* we pray. Still, I hear it a lot. "I don't know where to start. I don't know how to pray."

So let me offer you an old, but powerful tool for your prayer life. This formula will help to keep your prayers balanced and on point. Try it now, and record your thoughts below.

It's called ACTS (as in the Book of Acts in the Bible). There are four parts to this prayer.

Adoration—Begin your prayer by expressing adoration to God for who he is. Focus on his character and attributes. Praise him for who he is.

Confession—Confess your sin to God, but more importantly, express your *sins*. Be specific. List your sins before the Lord, and ask him to forgive each one.

Thanksgiving—This is different from adoration. Rather than praising God for *who he is* (adoration), here you will thank God for *what he's done*. Be specific. Write out the things you are thankful for today.

Supplication—Now do what you already do when you pray, most times. Ask God for something. Ask for his blessings, wisdom, and healing. Pray for his intervention in your life, and pray for others.

It's time to pray! Write down the specifics of this prayer.

Adoration: _____

_____

Confession: _____

_____

Tanksgiving: _____

_____

Supplication: _____

_____

Day 1
Knock Three Times

Before Jesus got out of the first chapter of Mark, we read this: "Very early in the morning, while it was still dark, Jesus got up, left the house and went off to a solitary place, where he prayed" (Mark 1:35).

What we do in the morning matters. What mattered to Jesus? It's pretty clear. He prayed—early and often.

If you suffer from porn or sex addiction, I know this. If you could overcome this on your own, you already would have. Now it's time to tap into your Higher Power. And there is no better way to do that than through prayer. Don't just pray a little. An old song says, "Knock three times." Pray like that. Seek God at least three times each day.

Charles Spurgeon called prayer "a spiritual transaction with the Creator of Heaven and Earth." Oswald Chambers wrote, "It's not so much that prayer changes things, but that prayer changes me."

Porn addicts are like the boy possessed by a demon. Jesus said the demon could be cast out, but "this kind can come out only by prayer" (Mark 9:29).

If you are tired of battling the demons, it's time to pray. If you have sought freedom in your own strength, it's time to pray. If you have tried therapy, the 12 Steps, and reading a pile of materials, but have still come up short—it's time to pray.

Day 2
Pray

"Pray continually" (1 Thessalonians 5:17).

You won't find a more straightforward verse than that one.

Unfortunately, too many of us pray too little. A report by *Newsweek* concluded that 91 percent of women pray, as well as 85 percent of men. That number rises to 100 percent among golfers once they reach the green. But most limit their prayers to quickies before a difficult putt or questionable meal.

For most of us, serious prayer is relegated to times of crisis. We are like the girl who prayed after taking a test in school: "God, either make Boston the capital of Vermont or lose my test paper by tomorrow morning."

Like that girl, we all face tests—especially those of us engaged in a fight for purity. We need to live like a mountain climber. When the wind comes against him, he gets on his knees.

Are the winds of temptation threatening to blow you off course? Then get on your knees today.

Robert Kennedy said, "All of us might wish at times that we lived in a more tranquil world, but we don't. And if our times are difficult and perplexing, so are they challenging and filled with opportunity."

The trials you face today are filled with opportunity—to grow, rely on God, and turn to him in prayer.

Day 3
Production Without Passion

God did not create human doings, but human beings. He is far more concerned with what is happening *in* you than what is happening *around* you or being accomplished *by* you. He is not looking for production, but passion.

Oswald Chambers wrote, "The greatest competitor of devotion to Jesus is service for Jesus."

Speaking to a church that was doing all the right things, God said, "Yet I hold this against you. You have forsaken the love you had at first" (Revelation 2:4).

We live in busy times. We fill our schedules with things that are all good, but God gets left out. In the story of Mary and Martha, we see two sisters seeking to please God in their own way. One gave Jesus her effort while the other gave Jesus her heart. And that was the sister most blessed.

God longs for you to spend time with him. Read a few verses of Scripture, talk to him as a friend, and just sit in his presence. Set down your phone and pick up your Bible. Get off your computer and get on your knees.

I love the way John Piper said it. "One of the greatest uses of Twitter and Facebook will be to prove at the Last Day that prayerlessness was not from lack of time."

Forget about production and focus on passion. If you get your passion right, the production will take care of itself.

Day 4
Dark Clouds

C.S. Lewis called pain "God's great unwanted gift." Nothing brings more pain than losing our sobriety. The disappointment, shame, and guilt can feel overwhelming. In those moments we feel all alone. Even God has left us.

Or has he?

There is an interesting verse tucked away in one of the least read books of the Bible. At a time when King Solomon and the Israelites were facing a bleak future—largely due to their own poor decisions—the Bible says, "God spoke from a dark cloud" (2 Chronicles 6:1).

It's easy to see God in a sunrise or sunset. It's easy to feel his presence on a mountain, by a stream, or on the beach. When the choir hits the high note, when the preacher hits a home run, and when we experience showers of blessing, we see, hear, and touch God.

But what about in the hard times? Hear it again: "God spoke from a *dark* cloud."

Here's the good news. If the storm clouds have gathered, if the pain is massive, and if sobriety seems elusive, God is still there. When recovery seems to be no more than a mirage in the desert, God is still speaking.

So don't wait for the sunshine to return, for times to get better, or for sobriety to come easy. Listen for God's voice *now*; seek his face *now*; lean into Him *now*. Claim one of the Bible's great promises. *"God spoke from a dark cloud."*

Day 5
Antidote to Anxiety

Paul gave the church only two options. "Do not be anxious about anything, but in everything by prayer and supplication make your requests known to God" (Philippians 4:6).

You can worry. Or you can pray. Pick one.

The Anxiety and Depression Association of America states, "Anxiety disorders are the most common mental illness in the U.S., affecting 40 million adults in the United States, or 18.1 percent of the population. Yet, only 36.9 percent of those suffering receive treatment."

But anxiety is not new. Famed 19th century preacher Charles Spurgeon said of anxiety, "Anxiety does not empty tomorrow of its sorrows, but only empties today of its strength."

And 21st century preacher Max Lucado offered this advice. "Become a worry-slapper. Treat frets like mosquitoes. Do you procrastinate when a bloodsucking bug lights on your skin? Of course you don't! You give the critter the slap it deserves. Be equally decisive with anxiety."

The great worry-slapper is prayer. To find victory, you must turn your hurts, habits, hang-ups, and anxiety over to God.

Day 6
Driving Out Your Demons

The second Gospel tells the story of a boy possessed by demons. His father brought him to Jesus' disciples in hope that they would cast out the demons. But they failed to do so. So the man brought his son to Jesus, who cast out the demons. The disciples asked Jesus why they had failed in their efforts. Jesus offered a simple answer. "This kind can come out only by prayer" (Mark 9:29).

"Only by prayer," Jesus said.

Perhaps you can identify with the boy in this story. You feel like there is something inside of you that has a craving for which there is no answer. You have tried to overcome your addiction in many ways. At first, you ignored it. Then you downplayed it. Eventually, you came to recognize it as the adversary that it is. But you still didn't understand that this is a spiritual battle.

It's time to do what the disciples did. It's time to call in reinforcements, because "this kind can come out only by prayer." But the power isn't actually in the prayer; it's in the One to whom you pray.

Charles Spurgeon defined prayer like this: "True prayer is neither a mere mental exercise nor a vocal performance. It is far deeper than that—it is a spiritual transaction with the creator of heaven and earth."

If you recognize the nature of the opposition, you are ready to get well. It's time to pray.

You have worked as though it all depended upon you. Now pray as though it all depends upon God. Because it does.

Day 7
Far Away

Patrick Carnes writes, "Addicts can clearly know they need to stop, but still cannot. Despite the consequences, they continue high-risk behaviors. They become so obsessed with destructive behaviors that all their life priorities—children, work, values, family, hobbies, friends—are sacrificed for the behavior and the preoccupation that goes with it. The addiction becomes a way to escape or obliterate pain. The addict needs the behavior in order to feel normal."

Carnes nailed it. But for even the "worst" addict, there is hope. The Bible says, "But you also said that no matter how far away we were, we could turn to you and start obeying your laws" (Nehemiah 1:9).

I love those words: *"no matter how far away we were."*

You may be really far from God today. But know this—his hearing is excellent. He can hear your cry from the next room, the next building, or the next universe. You will never be so far from God that you are beyond his reach.

You can reach out to God today. You *should* reach out to God today. Good intentions are not enough. Like Ralph Waldo Emerson said, "Good thoughts are no better than good dreams if you don't follow through."

Week 34
Routine

"I try to just focus on being in the same
routine every single day."

- Patrick Mahomes

THIS WEEK'S EXERCISE
Plan a Routine

Practice makes perfect.

When I was 15, my Dad took me to the local miniature golf course every day on his way to work. I spent all of my allowance playing miniature golf that summer. By August, I got really good. I set the course record with a 27 (par 36), and won enough tournaments that I no longer had to pay to play. (With each tournament win came several free passes.) By the end of the summer, I had worked my way up the ranks into the adult division, and qualified for the state tournament. I finished in 4th place in the Texas State Putt-Putt Championship, sponsored by Coca Cola. I only missed 1st place by three strokes.

Practice makes perfect.

Yes, the Putt-Putt story is real. I still have a 3-inch trophy somewhere as proof. But aside from bragging on the greatest athletic achievement of my life, let me repeat the bigger point.

Practice makes perfect.

That is true when mastering a musical instrument, excelling academically, or reaching one's full potential in sports that are every bit as demanding as miniature golf.

And in recovery—practice makes perfect.

This week, focus on one recovery activity. Do it over and over. Make it a daily priority. Set a time and place to focus on this recovery activity. Some examples you might choose from are listed here:

- Read recovery material (this book will do)
- Pray
- Make a call
- Meditate
- Memorize the 3rd Step Prayer
- Journal

Set a time and place each day so you can be consistent. Commit to this daily activity. Make it a daily routine. Write your routine below, then stick to it every day this week.

My daily activity: _____

_____

Day I will begin: _____

Place I will do this activity: _____

Time for this daily activity: _____

Check each day you follow this routine:

Day 1 _____

Day 2 _____

Day 3 _____

Day 4 _____

Day 5 _____

Day 6 _____

Day 7 _____

Day 1
In with the Old

Speaking of living the Christian life, G.K. Chesterton said, "The Christian ideal has not been tried and found wanting; it has been found difficult and left untried."

The same can be said of working the 12 Steps. The reason so many fail to find sobriety is not that the Steps don't work, but that they don't work the Steps. Israel's third king said it like this: "Whatever your hand finds to do, do it with all your might" (Ecclesiastes 9:10).

Vince Lombardi was right: "The price of success is hard work, dedication to the job at hand, and the determination that whether we win or lose, we have applied the best of ourselves to the task at hand."

If you are struggling to maintain sobriety, the key probably isn't reading a new book, finding a new therapist, or joining a new group. The key is working the old steps, committing to old principles, and staying with your old group.

Your problem isn't that you don't know enough, but that you don't do enough. But that can all change, starting today.

There is no silver bullet to recovery. It's about doing the same things that have always worked, one day at a time. You can start that process right now.

Day 2
Winning the Gold

In 2018, the Winter Olympics were hosted by South Korea. For the next 17 days the city of PyeongChang and surrounding areas played host to the world's greatest athletes, representing 90 countries and competing in 102 different events.

The United States sent 240 athletes to compete. Among them was Shani Davis, the 35-year-old speed skater from Chicago, who was the first black skater to win gold. Winner of 13 medals from the past three Winter Games, Davis explained the key to his enduring success with one word—"discipline."

Recovery is not a single event. And past success is no guarantee of future sobriety. We must keep competing—every day. Davis was successful at the Winter Games, in full sight of millions of viewers, because he had been hard at work for years, when no one was watching.

It's what you do when no one is watching that will keep you sober for today. Using the athletic metaphor, Paul told young Timothy, "Athletes cannot win the prize unless they follow the rules" (2 Timothy 2:5). There is no short cut to success. There are exercises to be done and rules to be followed. In recovery, we must maintain a regimen of disciplined activities. Recovery does not come easily, nor does it come quickly. But it does come, if we work at it.

Make a commitment today to the daily disciplines that will keep you sober.

Day 3
Stay the Course

Journalist Stewart Alsop wrote about his conversation with Winston Churchill in 1973. He related that the British Prime Minister had pondered, at the close of World War II, "America, it is a great and strong country, like a workhorse pulling the rest of the world out of despair. But will it stay the course?"

"Stay the course" would become a popular phrase for Presidents Ronald Reagan and George H.W. Bush.

Paul said it like this: "Let us not get tired of doing good, for we will reap at the proper time if we don't give up" (Galatians 6:9).

In recovery, it is so easy to give up. I've seen it happen far too often. First, they miss a few meetings. Then they quit working the 12 Steps, going to church, and connecting with others. Predictably, relapse occurs.

If you have started the journey to real sobriety, I offer three words: "Stay the course." If you are tempted to let up or give up, I say, "Stay the course." If you are tired of all the recovery work, I repeat, "Stay the course."

You know the things that work, the things you need to do. So keep doing them. Determine today, to stay the course.

Day 4
The Pareto Principle

Joseph Juran, the management expert who lived 103 years, is credited for initiating the 80/20 rule, also known as the law of the vital few or the principle of factor sparsity. The principle holds that roughly 80% of the effects in life result from 20% of the causes.

Juran named this principle after Italian economist Vilfredo Pareto, who taught the 80/20 connection while teaching at the University of Lausanne in 1896. Pareto noted that 80% of the land in Italy was owned by 20% of the population.

From that we have the Pareto Principle.

The Pareto Principle encapsulates the work of recovery. You will likely find that 20% of your efforts will produce 80% of your results. The lesson? Focus on a few things, and do them well.

One day, the Bible says, there was "a woman in the crowd who had suffered for twelve years with constant bleeding, and she could not find a cure. Coming up behind Jesus, she touched the fringe of his robe. Immediately, the bleeding stopped" (Luke 8:43-44).

The cure for a porn habit, sexting, or other forms of acting out, is not to do a bunch of good things okay. The cure is to do a few things really well.

Apply the Pareto Principle to recovery. Focus on just a few recovery activities. Then go all in with all you have.

Day 5
Holy Habits

Baseball Hall-of-Famer Al Kaline said, "You've got to develop good habits before the season begins. That way when the big play comes—and you never know when that will be—you will be ready."

Your sobriety tomorrow will be determined by what you do today. It's all about developing the right habits.

Camel Cigarettes knew this 50 years ago. They came out with an ad, in which they invited people to take the "30-day test." They asked people to try Camel for 30 days, knowing that by that time, they would be both loyal and addicted.

There was a man in the Bible who was the master of holy habits. His name was Daniel. When he was thrown to the lion's den, the king said, "May your God, whom you serve continually, rescue you!" (Daniel 6:16). King Darius had observed Daniel "distinguish himself by his exceptional qualities" (6:3) for 30 days—and longer. And it was the character developed by those habits—such as praying three times a day at the same place and time—that saw Daniel through.

Gandhi said, "Your actions become your habits, your habits become your values, and your values become your destiny."

Do you want sobriety tomorrow? Then develop holy habits today—prayer, Scripture reading, worship, meetings, recovery work. The more you do the right thing today, the harder it will be to do the wrong thing tomorrow.

Start developing one holy habit today in order to find real recovery tomorrow.

Day 6
Safe Travels

Jesus said, "Blessed are the pure in heart, for they will see God" (Matthew 5:8).

When we are in our general routine, staying pure is not as hard. But when we are out of our normal environment, temptations rise. It is critical that we commit to the battle for purity every hour, every day, all the time—especially when we travel.

Ruben Castaneda wrote a column for *U.S. News* on February 8, 2017, in which he offered 11 practical strategies for staying sober while traveling. These are some of those tips.

1. Plan ahead.
2. Make local contacts.
3. Bring recovery literature or recordings.
4. Remember your H.A.L.T.
5. Stay in contact with your home network.
6. Remove as many temptations as possible.
7. Avoid certain people and places.
8. Keep to your routine.

There is no battle more important than the one for purity. That is why Jesus offered this special promise just for the pure in heart—that "they will see God." Prepare for that battle—especially when you are away from home.

Apply the eight tips listed above the next time you go out of town.

Day 7
It Takes 90 Days

It's time to grow up.

Paula Poundstone said, "Adults are always asking kids what they want to be when they grow up because they are looking for ideas."

Paul wrote, "When I was a child, I spoke like a child, I thought like a child, I reasoned like a child. When I became a man, I gave up childish ways" (1 Corinthians 13:11).

For the porn addict, growing up takes time—*about 90 days*.

T.J. Nelson says that brain scans show that with any addictive substance (including porn) it takes 90–100 days for your midbrain to start forming connections with your frontal lobe. This means if you make it to 90 days of sobriety, your chances for long-term success skyrockets. Nelson concludes, "Therefore, your primary goal should be to do whatever it takes to make it to 90 days. Then you'll be able to stay away from it long-term to the point that after a few years your brain has healed itself."

Norman Doidge writes, in *The Brain that Changes Itself*, "Once porn is left behind, the brain pathways it created will start to fade."

The evidence is in. To find a lifetime of recovery, you need to find 90 days of recovery. That is why we have written the ***90-Day Recovery Guide***.

Week 35
Worship

"God made and governs the world. He has commanded us to love and worship him and no other."

- Isaac Newton

THIS WEEK'S EXERCISE
Listen to 'Flawless'

In 2014, MercyMe came out with what has become my favorite song of this millennium. It's called *Flawless*. The song won the GMA Dove Award for Song of the Year and sat atop the charts for several weeks.

I love this line from the song:

"No matter the bumps, no matter the bruises, no matter the scars, still the truth is, The cross has made, the cross has made you flawless."

Bart Millard, lead singer, gives us the story behind the song. "Christ looks at you and says, 'You are the most amazing thing I've ever seen. In that sense, you are flawless.'"

Worship should be a frequent component of your recovery plan. Here's a great way to enter into worship this week. Listen to the song *Flawless*, then journal on how this song impacted you and spoke to your recovery.

You can easily find the song on YouTube. If you don't know how to do that, find anyone under 35, and they can help you! Listen to the song three times before you journal.

Date I listened to the song: _____

What this song says about God's grace: _____

_____

_____

_____

What this song says about my recovery: _____

_____

_____

_____

Day 1
The Saw

A man had a firewood factory that employed hundreds of men. He paid them well and gave them specific directions on what to do. But their work was slow and unproductive. Eventually, he had no choice. He fired the men and purchased a circular saw powered by a gas engine. In one hour, the new saw accomplished more than all the other men had done in a week.

The man asked his new saw. "How can you turn out so much work? Are you sharper than the saws my men were using before?"

The saw responded, "No, I am not sharper than the other saws. The difference is the gas engine. I have a stronger power behind me. I am productive because of the power that is working through me, not because my blade is stronger."

The man or woman who finds successful recovery doesn't do so because he or she has a sharper blade. It's all about the power within. The Bible calls that power the Holy Spirit.

Jesus promised his earliest followers, "You will receive power when the Holy Spirit comes on you" (Acts 1:8).

That's the secret. It's not the sharpness of the saw, but the presence of the Spirit.

Ask God to empower your saw through the filling and power of the Holy Spirit.

Day 2
Seeing God

Isaiah has a book of the Bible that bears his name, but he was a common man. While he likely had wealth and was the most influential prophet of his time, he was a man of the people. Despite his achievements in ministry, he stood before God in fear. He recorded the following experience.

"Then one of the seraphim flew to me with a live coal in his hand, which he had taken with tongs from the altar. With it he touched my mouth and said, 'See, this has touched your lips; your guilt is taken away and your sin is now atoned for'" (Isaiah 6:6-7).

Isaiah stood before the Lord in awe, unsure of what to do next. Then, when God called him to go minister among his people, he was ready. "Here I am. Send me!" (6:8).

Any true encounter with God changes what comes next. The same is true in recovery. The best medicine for the disease of addiction is an encounter with the God of the universe.

John Piper writes, "In the end the heart longs not for any of God's good gifts, but for God himself. To see him and know him and be in his presence is the soul's final feast. Beyond this there is no quest."

Try this for today. Rather than seeking recovery, seek God.

Day 3
Power in Praise

There is power in praising God.

The final Book says, "All the angels stood around the throne singing, 'Blessing and glory and honor and power and strength be to our God forever and ever!'" (Revelation 7:12).

In his message on praise, Tony Evans said, "If you're facing difficulty of any kind or size, begin to sing songs of praise to the Lord, and you will see your enemies defeated. Not only that, but your heart will be lifted, and you will sense a peace inside like nothing you have known. God wants to restore the peace you have lost. If you will let him, he will give you a fresh touch of his peace, love, and grace when you praise him."

Pastor Todd Gaddis lists seven reasons to praise God: (a) the Bible commands it, (b) praise facilitates access to God, (c) praise is where God lives, (d) praise promotes productivity, (e) praise chases away despair, (f) praise is an effective weapon against the devil, and (g) God is worthy of your praise.

Let me add an eighth reason to praise God. In your lowest moment, at your darkest hour, God was there—ready to scoop you up, lift you up, clean you up, and point you in a whole new direction. You have much to praise God for. Now's as good a time as any to get started.

Take a moment now and praise God. That's all the direction you need.

Day 4
Frankenstein

Frankenstein is one of the most enduring movies of all-time. The most remembered lines of this 1931 film are the words of Dr. Frankenstein, spoken when his monster began to move. "It's alive! It's alive!"

The original line was a bit different: "It's alive! It's alive! In the name of God! Now I know what it's like to be God!"

Censors cut the "God" part of Frankenstein's words, feeling they were sacrilege.

The original words of this crazy doctor represent the heart of us all. The first temptation of man was that he might "be like God" (Genesis 3:5).

We sink into the depths of sex addiction when we take on the role of God—deciding what is best for us.

Research conducted by Matthew Killingsworth and Daniel Gilbert of Harvard University traces the search for happiness in the heart of man. Reported by the journal *Science*, the study concluded that men and women engage in improper sexual activities in search of control and fulfillment. For many, this is the closest experience to becoming like God.

Like Frankenstein's monster, you can come alive. But you can only experience the freedom God has for you when you quit living a self-absorbed life in an attempt to be like God.

Day 5
Outburst of the Soul

"David sang to the Lord when he was delivered from the hand of all his enemies and from the hand of Saul" (2 Samuel 22:1).

The people who surrounded King David grew accustomed to his musical outbursts. It was David who danced "before the Lord with all his might" (2 Samuel 6:14). It was David who was the most prolific songwriter of the Bible.

Nineteenth century English composer Frederick Delius said, "Music is the outburst of the soul."

The Scriptures reverberate with the songs of people who were enraptured by God's work. Moses and Miriam harmonized praise after God had led his people out of Egypt (Exodus 15). Solomon crooned his way through the Song of Songs, celebrating marriage. Isaiah offered a song of praise from the coming choir of the new Jerusalem (Isaiah 26:1).

You can go to counseling and 12-Step groups for years and never hear this advice—*Sing more!*

The biblical record offers overwhelming support for the notion that singing to the Lord brings incredible benefits. Praise engages the spirit and ignites the soul. It raises your eyes to the heavenlies, fills your heart with hope, and opens heaven's doors.

Delius was right. "Music is the outburst of the soul." It worked for David. It will work for you.

It's time for an outburst of your soul. Lift your heart and voice to the Lord. Find time—today—to sing praises to your King.

Day 6
A Chance Encounter

"Sweet hour of prayer,
Sweet hour of prayer,
That calls me from a world of care,
And bids me at my Father's throne
Make all my wants and wishes known.
In seasons of distress and grief
My soul has often found relief.
And oft escaped the tempter's snare
By thy return, sweet hour of prayer."

A better hymn was never written. But we almost didn't get to see this iconic work.

William W. Walford, an obscure, blind lay preacher, owned a small shop in England. In his spare time, he composed poems for his personal devotions. In his mind, he wrote the words above and committed them to memory. A friend named Thomas Salmon stopped by his shop one day in 1842. Walford asked Salmon if he'd write down his new poem.

Three years later, Salmon passed the poem on to the editor of the *New York Observer*, who printed it on September 13, 1845. A local composer named William B. Bradbury saw it and wrote the tune. The result is the hymn we still sing today.

Sadly, Walford died before his poem was put to song. He never saw the results of his labor.

Like Walford, this side of heaven, you may never see the impact your words have on others. You will say about 7,000 words today. Make them count.

"God works in you, both to will and to work for his good pleasure" (Philippians 2:13). God will use your words, your story, and every "chance encounter" in ways you can't imagine—if you only submit to him.

Day 7
A Singing English Teacher

In a sea of forgotten middle school teachers, one still sticks in my head. His name was Elga Steward. I still remember the very first day of class. While we were all seated at our desks, Mr. Steward was nowhere to be seen. Then we heard him before we saw him. With a booming baritone voice, he came down the hall singing the words to *Invictus*, by William Henley. The first stanza follows.

"Out of the night that covers me,
Black as the pit from pole to pole,
I thank whatever gods may be
For my unconquerable soul."

Catch that first line: *"Out of the night that covers me."* This is the life of an addict. We live in the shadows, both literally and figuratively. Pornography loves the darkness. I tell clients, "The opposite of recovery is not addiction, but secrecy."

To get well, you must emerge from the "night that covers" you. A good place to start is with a personal walk with Christ, "the light that shines in darkness" (John 1:5).

Flee the night that covers you and embrace the light, as that is the only way you will get well.

Week 36
Lust

"I've looked on many women with lust. I've committed adultery in my heart many times."

\- Jimmy Carter

THIS WEEK'S EXERCISE
List Your Lust

Financial freedom experts like Dave Ramsey all suggest that before a person can get out of debt, he needs to know where he is spending his money. Clients are encouraged to journal for 30 days, to record all of their expenses. With that information, they can begin to put together a realistic budget.

The same idea applies to recovery. Whether you are trying to recover from a load of debt or a load of improper sexual activity, you need to know how bad the problem really is.

I love the SA definition of sobriety—achieving progressive victory over *lust*. If we only deal with our behaviors, we will never get well. The cycle of addiction tells us that we only do what we think. The genesis of acting out is lust. We must deal with our lust problem. But first, we have to measure the size and scope of that problem.

Max Dupree says the first job of every leader is to define reality as it really is. Likewise, the first task of the sex addict is to identify his struggle with lust as specifically as possible.

Ready for a painful and eye-opening exercise? List each occurrence of lust for the next seven days. You don't need to go into detail; just jot down a few words to identify the nature of each instance. Examples might be: "saw woman at the mall," "thought of a past partner," "lusted after woman on TV show," "objectified my wife."

Day 1

    a. _____

    b. _____

    C. _____

Day 2

    a. _____

    b. _____

    C. _____

Day 3

    a. _____

    b. _____

    C. _____

Day 4

    a. _____

    b. _____

    C. _____

Day 5

    a. _____

    b. _____

    C. _____

Day 6

    a. _____

    b. _____

    C. _____

Day 7

    a. _____

    b. _____

    C. _____

Day 1
Pet Anaconda

Fred thought he had a good idea.

His love for pets started out with goldfish, then escalated to birds. Before he knew it, his addiction progressed to cats, and then dogs. But that still wasn't enough to satisfy Fred. He always found himself wanting that next pet, the one that would finally satisfy his need for animal companionship.

So Fred bought an anaconda. An anaconda is a snake. A big snake. A hungry snake.

As long as the anaconda was in its cage, all was fine. But one time (with snakes it only takes one time), Fred left the cage door open—just a little bit. And then he went to bed.

How does this story end? Well, let's just say that old Fred didn't wake up the next day to his wife, but to his Savior.

The point of the story tells itself. Let's give your anaconda a name—pornography. You think you can stay safe by keeping it locked up, out of sight, or on the computer. But just one time (with porn it only takes one time), it escapes from the pages or computer into your memory banks.

And then it's over. You never had a chance.

Like the anaconda, we often don't see the threat of porn or sex addiction until "our sin sweeps us away" (Isaiah 64:6). Don't give one inch to temptation; it never ends well.

Day 2
L.U.S.T.

I recently read the following account, as told by counselor Dwight Bain.

"Sarah woke up from a deep sleep at 3 a.m. and realized that her husband wasn't in bed, so she got up to see if he was okay. She was not prepared for what she saw next. Her husband of 27 years, whom she respected as a man of integrity, was sitting in front of their home computer in a trance, while looking at the most sexually graphic pictures that she had ever seen. She asked him what he was doing. His response—'I don't know.'"

To win the victory over sex addiction, we must win the victory over lust. In fact, Sexaholics Anonymous defines sobriety that way: "progressive victory over lust."

Where does lust come from? Let me offer this simple formula to keep in mind.

- L = Lonely
- U = Unfulfilled
- S = Stressed
- T = Tired

When you are lonely, unfulfilled, stressed, or tired, lust is lurking around the corner. The next thing you know, you will find yourself confronted with some uncomfortable questions, for which you won't have any better answers than—"I don't know."

Day 3
The Untold Price We Pay

The Bible tells the story of a man named Amnon who fell in love with Tamar, his half sister (2 Samuel 13). Here we find the progressive nature of addiction. What Amnon took in with his eyes became lust. Lust led to fantasy, which resulted in acting out.

Then we discover the final chapter in every episode of acting out. Amnon's brief moment of ecstasy was followed by an overwhelming sense of shame. What happened in Amnon's life is the story of every addict. He wanted what he shouldn't have and didn't want it once he had it.

Immediately after he committed his sin, "Suddenly Amnon's love turned to hate, and he hated her even more than he had loved her" (13:15). Amnon became a permanent wreck. Amnon discovered a hard truth: the one thing more painful than not feeding our lust is feeding our lust.

The next time you fantasize about crossing the boundaries God has put in place, pause just long enough to play out the end of the story in your head. It never ends well.

When you do cross those lines, even if just in your head, keep the words of Watchman Nee close by. "Now is the hour we should humbly prostrate ourselves before God, willing to be convinced afresh of our sins by the Holy Spirit."

Day 4
Living at Disney World

The September 20, 2019, edition of *USA Today* included an interesting story about the Golden Oak—a gated community of a few dozen homes in Orlando. They start at $2.5 million. What makes the Golden Oak special? Every house is built on the grounds of Disney World.

For some, visiting Disney is not enough. They want to live there. Life is defined by the next show or ride.

This is a picture of modern marriage. Feeling unfulfilled by their marriage, spouses think they will be happy if they can just move into Disney World:

1. Fantasyland—escape from the real world
2. Tomorrowland—escape from the present world
3. Adventureland—escape from the predictable world
4. Frontierland—escape from the former world

Life is one ride after the next. Eventually, even the most exhilarating of rides becomes too familiar. So we move on to the next thrill, convinced that there must be a new ride out there that will hold our interest.

One of the things we like most is that Disney World makes no demands of us, beyond a Season Pass, at most. If, at the end of the year, we are still having fun, we can sign up for another year. If not, well, that's why God created Busch Gardens and Six Flags.

The Bible warns, "Whoever loves pleasure will be a poor man" (Proverbs 21:17). How does this work? In simple terms, the person (husband or wife) who puts personal pleasure ahead of his or her partner will go bankrupt in an endless and fruitless search for the real thing.

Your "ride" may be an addiction, or some other form of pleasure. May I suggest, it's time to join the real world.

Day 5
Can God Heal My Addiction—Now?

Can God heal your addiction right now? The short answer is "Yes." But the honest answer is "Probably not."

Of course, God *can*. But I'm not sure I've ever seen it happen. Of course, God can take a man with 50 years of addiction and immediately remove the urges. But here's the problem. For God to do that would require him to reconstruct the very brain he constructed in the first place.

Let me explain.

There is an old myth that it takes 21 days to break a habit. Actually, it takes 21 days to create a habit. And it takes 90 days for "the brain to reset itself and shake off the immediate influence of a drug," according to research conducted by *Time* magazine.

At Duffy's Napa Valley Rehab, they have found that, "Although 90 days is considered the gold standard of treatment, addiction is a life-long battle—even after years of sobriety."

The Bible says, "Many followed Jesus, and he healed them all" (Matthew 12:15). Sometimes that healing comes fast, but with a disease of the brain, it usually takes a lifetime.

But the first 90 days is critical. That's Why I wrote *A 90-Day Recovery Guide*. And that's why I take men through my 90-day program based on my book.

Can God remove your addiction immediately? Yes, he can. So here's my suggestion. Ask him now. And if he does remove all urges, praise him for that! But if the urge to act out is still there tomorrow, continue to engage this program of recovery.

Day 6
Private Thoughts

Stephen Arterburn has done the research. In *The Secrets Men Keep*, he reveals a study that he commissioned of 3,600 men on the subject of fantasy. His findings: 57 percent of men admit to "frequent and intense" sexual fantasies. Among self-identified Christians, the number is similar, at 54 percent. So what's the big thing about fantasy?

Gordon MacDonald offers answers, in his book, *When Men Think Private Thoughts*. MacDonald writes, "What nature or custom or circumstance denies or forbids, the imagination is likely to create." He continues, "If the fantasies are strong enough, they may lead to adultery or other immoral acts, as well as the breakup of a marriage."

For too many of us, fantasy is set up on the top shelf that never gets dusted. We know it's there, but we pretend it doesn't matter. Enter Solomon with these poignant words: "He who works his land will have abundant food, but the one who chases fantasies will have his fill of poverty" (Proverbs 28:19).

Let me translate that verse for you. Fantasies never fulfill. Indulging in fantasy is like quenching your thirst with salt water. The fantasy is never an end, but a means. It never satisfies. Indulging one's sexual fantasies disrupts sanity. Simply entertaining the fantasy will leave you frustrated and empty.

The answer? Quit chasing fantasy. Consume your thought life with healthier pursuits.

Fantasy is often the last battle an addict must fight. But you can win this battle—one thought at a time.

Day 7
Never Satisfied

Lust is progressive. It never satisfies. There's an old story about God's people returning from exile to Jerusalem. They started to rebuild the Temple, but when they faced opposition, they quit. In frustration, they turned inward, building lavish homes for themselves instead of furnishing God's House. For them, life was about taking the easy path and indulging in the pleasure of the moment.

In stepped a prophet named Haggai. He wrote, "Look what's happening to you! You have planted much but harvested little. You eat but are not satisfied. You drink but are still thirsty" (Haggai 1:5-6).

That is the picture of every addict. We eat, but are still hungry. We drink, but are still thirsty. There's a reason for this.

We are chasing temporary solutions to permanent problems.

I have acid reflux. It causes a burning in my esophagus. Sometimes, I do the right thing and drink a disgusting tasting liquid before bed. And I sleep all night. But other times, I eat a bowl of ice cream. Why? Because it tastes better in the moment. And it actually coats my throat, so it feels better for a few minutes. The problem is that in four or five hours, the pain returns and I end up having to drink the medicine anyway.

Every day, we are tempted to drink in the lust. And it feels good in the moment. But it only masks the real pain. What's the solution? Drink of the Living Water that never runs dry.

Week 37
Sowing

"Even after a bad harvest there must be sowing."

- Seneca

THIS WEEK'S EXERCISE
Do a Random Act

The ultimate example of biblical giving is doing something for someone who cannot repay you, and while receiving no credit for your actions.

This week's focus will be sowing good seeds of recovery. You must invest your time and attention today in what you want to become tomorrow. This principle applies to all facets of the Christian life.

This week's exercise will call on you to sow a seed into the life of another person who cannot repay you. It's called a random act of kindness. There are many ways you can do this. Consider a few examples.

- Buy a recovery book for someone in your 12-Step group.
- Make a call to a friend who is new to recovery.
- Buy an inexpensive gift card for your sponsor.
- Do something kind for someone whom you have injured in the past.
- Send a small gift to a recovery ministry. (*There's Still Hope* accepts large gifts, as well!)
- Help set up for a meeting at your church this week.
- Bake cookies for a neighbor.
- Visit someone in a nursing home.

There is no limit to the things you can do to sow seeds of recovery. The amazing thing about recovery is that the more you give, the more you get back. Seeds are small, but they can make a huge difference in the life of the recipient—and the giver.

What will you do this week to sow a seed of recovery? _____

_____

_____

Day 1
Universal Principle

There is a universal principle that applies to addiction. It's called sowing and reaping. The ancient prophet Hosea said, "Plant the good seeds of righteousness, and you will harvest a crop of love" (Hosea 10:12).

The mistake most of us make is that we want good results without doing the things that produce those results. We want the blessing of the crop without the pain of the work.

Muhammad Ali said, "The crown is never won in the ring. It's just recognized there. The crown is won on the streets, where I run miles when no one is watching, and in the gym, where I put my body through hell so I will be ready to go 15 rounds."

Recovery is never won in the first round. You have to go the distance. But tomorrow's victory is decided by today's work. If you want to be well tomorrow you need to pray today. If you want to be strong tomorrow, go to a meeting tonight. If you want to see a good harvest, start planting seeds now.

Pete Rose, baseball's all-time hit king, said, "My father taught me that the only way you can make good at anything is to practice, and then practice some more." Jackson Brown said, "You can't hire someone to practice for you."

Everything significant that happens to you tomorrow will have already been determined by the things you did today. What you sow today you will reap tomorrow. That is a universal principle of life.

Day 2
Winning Tomorrow's Sobriety Today

I owe today's sobriety to the actions of yesterday. Tomorrow's sobriety remains unfinished business. Let's finish Hosea's quote from yesterday's lesson: "Break up your unplowed ground; for it is time to seek the Lord, until he comes and showers his righteousness on you" (Hosea 10:12).

The fruit we reap tomorrow will mostly be determined by the time we go to bed tonight. What we sow today, we will reap tomorrow. Matthew Henry wrote, "Every action is seed sown." And it cuts both ways.

The key, Hosea said, is to "break up your unplowed ground." That means to spend serious time with God, asking him to soften our hearts, to unearth that which we have buried deep beneath the rocky soil. And then we plant new seeds, knowing that no seed is too small.

C.S. Lewis wrote, in *Mere Christianity*, "The smallest good act today is the capture of a strategic point from which, a few months later, you may be able to go on to victories you never dreamed of. And an apparently trivial indulgence in lust may launch an attack otherwise impossible."

Today, you have two choices. You can ask God to soften your heart and then do a "good act." Or you can surrender to "an apparently trivial indulgence of lust." And either way, you will probably be okay for today.

But tomorrow's another story. Today you make your choices. Tomorrow your choices will make you. Every action is seed sown.

Day 3
Jumping Fleas

There was a study done on fleas. Researchers put fleas into a container and then put a lid on the top. The fleas immediately tried to jump out, but they hit the lid again and again. Before long, they realized they were stuck. At one point the researchers removed the lid, but to their surprise, the fleas didn't try to jump out anymore. They had hit that lid so many times they had become conditioned to thinking they couldn't get out. Even though the lid was off, they didn't even try to jump out.

Like those fleas, many of us have grown so accustomed to our failure that we have quit trying to jump out of our box. We have accepted lives within the box of pornography, masturbation, and affairs. Because our half-hearted attempts at sobriety have failed us, we've quit trying.

We need to dream again. We need to dream of a life free of the loneliness, pain, and addiction. And that's where God steps in. He is the creator of dreams. He has promised us that "young men shall see visions, and old men will dream dreams" (Acts 2:17).

God spoke to men in dreams throughout Scripture. Here are just a few examples: King Saul (1 Samuel 28:15), Daniel (Daniel 1:17), Abimelek (Genesis 20:3), Joseph (Matthew 2:13), God's children (Numbers 12:6), old men (Joel 2:28), and Job (Job 33:15).

Foreign correspondent Claude M. Bristol said simply, "You have to think big to be big."

If you are to ever escape your box, you'll have to think large, dream big, and jump high. Are you ready to leave the box? Then ask God for a new dream.

Day 4
Children

Children are pursuing porn at earlier ages than ever. A technology company called Bitdefender has found that of all who view porn under the age of 18, 22 percent of those are age nine or under.

Sadly, children often step into porn—and other addictions—because of their parents. Harvard Medical School has concluded that "children whose parents abuse alcohol face significantly higher risks of medical and behavioral problems, including substance abuse."

A 2016 study conducted by Michigan State University found that "a father's psychological well-being significantly influences the well-being of his child."

Net Nanny has concluded that the single most significant influence on a child's sexual behavior is that of his or her parents. The key to raising porn-free kids, they said in their 2017 study, is to "model positive behavior you want your child to emulate."

The fact is, you reproduce who you are, not who you want.

It's never too early to start. The Bible says to take God's standards and "impress them on your children" (Deuteronomy 6:7).

Stacia Tauscher was right when she wrote, "We worry about what a child will become tomorrow, yet we forget that he is someone today."

If you have a child, today is the best day to start becoming the parent she needs you to be.

Day 5
A Little Seed

"Will I ever get it?" "Will recovery ever stick?" "When the temptation hits, how will I know if I have what it takes to stay strong?"

I hear these questions all the time. Fortunately, we have an answer—from the lips of Jesus.

"Jesus said, 'The Kingdom of God is like a farmer who scatters seed on the ground. Night and day, while he's asleep or awake, the seed sprouts and grows, but he does not understand how it happens'" (Mark 4:26-27).

The farmer spreads his seed, then God takes over. The same principle works in recovery. If you take the actions of recovery, God will do a work that you cannot see. But when the battle hits, you will find that you have what it takes to win.

I do five miles a day on the treadmill. When I'm done, I get off right where I started. I haven't really gone anywhere. But the benefits are still there—better conditioning, more energy, and sore feet! Exercise today brings benefits tomorrow.

od took an orphan named Esther and put her in the right position to save his people. She didn't realize it at the time, but God was at work in her, to perform a higher purpose.

Joel Osteen says, "At this very moment, God is working behind the scenes in your life, arranging things in your favor."

Plant the seeds of recovery today, and you will be amazed at what God will do in your life—even when you don't see it.

Day 6
Job Reversal

God says we always reap what we have sown. Even after we have been forgiven, we must deal with the consequences of our actions. It may take considerable time to finish harvesting the negative consequences of our past.

Charles Stanley says it like this: "Rebellion against God always has a consequence of some sort, even if it's only guilt."

But the law of planting and harvesting can work to our benefit, as well. Paul said, "The point is this: whoever sows sparingly will also reap sparingly, and whoever sows bountifully will also reap bountifully" (2 Corinthians 9:6).

Henry David Thoreau wrote, "Goodness is the only investment that never fails."

Where most of us get off the rails is in reversing roles with God. We act as though he is to plant the seeds of preferred circumstances and blessing, while we do the work of harvesting. The opposite is true. If we do the work of planting through spiritual disciplines and recovery work, God will bring a harvest of blessing we could otherwise never know.

Day 7
The Price Is Right

On November 22, 1963, shots rang out in Dallas. We are still reaping the consequences today.

Solomon wrote, "A wicked person earns deceptive wages, but the one who sows righteousness reaps a sure reward" (Proverbs 11:18).

God says we always reap what we have sown. Even after we have been forgiven, we must deal with the consequences of what we have done. It may take time to finish harvesting the negative consequences of our actions and past sins. But know this—the harvest will come.

Stephen Covey is right: "While we are free to choose our actions, we are not free to choose the consequences of our actions."

Robert Louis Stevenson said it like this: "Everybody, sooner or later, will sit down to a banquet of consequences."

The reverse is also true. When you plant good seeds—such as making amends, giving back, and living a sober life—a positive harvest will follow.

The fact is, your actions today will reap a harvest for years to come. So plant carefully.

Week 38
Triggers

"I'm an actor who believes we all have triggers to any stage of emotion. It's not always easy to find, but it's still there."

\- Hugh Jackman

THIS WEEK'S EXERCISE
H.A.L.T.!

We all have triggers—people, places, or predicaments that put us at the brink of a relapse. But there are four specific triggers that AA has been talking about for years. This simple formula has found its way into recovery material of all kinds, and is often used by therapists.

We are most vulnerable when we are *hungry*, *angry*, *lonely*, or *tired*.

1. Hungry

This is obvious. When we go without food, we become agitated. Our chemistry is off, and we seek to self-medicate. We want quick gratification. And too often, we find that in sex, rather than food.

2. Angry

Anger is a huge component of addiction. When we are angry at someone, resentment builds up. Anger is destructive. When we are angry at someone—even if it seems justifiable at the time—it only hurts us. An angry person thinks he deserves pleasure to even the score. And too often, he finds this in sex.

3. Lonely

When we are lonely, we tend to isolate. That always spells trouble, because we only stay sober within community. Rarely does a person act out except when he is alone—and lonely.

4. Tired

When we are overworked and don't get enough rest, we let our defenses down. To maintain sobriety requires diligence. God has created us for rest. To not get enough rest is to break one of the commandments. And it puts our recovery at risk.

Pick an exercise.

Exercise #1—Rate your personal H.A.L.T.

Which of these are your biggest challenges: hungry, angry, lonely, tired?

_____

How are you tempted to act out by this trigger? _____

_____

_____

Exercise #2—People, places, predicaments

Give one example for each of these triggers in your personal life:
- People: _____
- Place: _____
- Predicament: _____

Day 1
"Danger, Will Robinson"

It was one of the great television shows of the 1960s—*Lost in Space*. Every Wednesday night from 1965 to 1968, I tuned in. If I missed *Lost in Space*, I lost my mind. For those of you younger than me (about 95% of the world), here's the synopsis. The show followed the ventures of the Robinsons, a pioneering family of space colonists who struggled to stay alive. CBS caught every moment.

Will Robinson was a teenage boy whose curiosity nearly cost him his life—in virtually every one of the 83 episodes. That's where the family robot came in. With three words, he steered Will from the clutches of death.

"Danger, Will Robinson."

We all need to hear that voice in our head—"Danger." When we begin to browse porn sites—"Danger!" When we go to certain dating sites—"Danger!" When we go to lunch with an attractive coworker—"Danger!" When we put ourselves in compromising situations—"Danger!"

We have this promise: "The Lord will guard your going out and your coming in" (Psalm 121:8). He often does this with a still, small voice.

Listen for that voice. Listen for his warning. Recognize his message.

"Danger!"

Are you putting yourself in a position of great temptation? Then heed the voice of God—"Danger, Will Robinson."

Day 2
Stress

Stress is not your friend.

The American Institute of Stress has identified 50 things stress will do to you, and none of them are good. These include headaches, backaches, neck aches, and toothaches. Stress causes stuttering and stammering, faintness and forgetfulness, blushing and belching, nausea and nightmares, constipation and confusion, diarrhea and depression, panic and pain.

Dr. Bessel Van Der Kolk wrote, "When you have stress, your body keeps score."

I heard about two high school buddies who had long since gone their separate ways. Seeing each other for the first time in 20 years, they met up at a high school reunion. One of the men said to his old friend, "I have to ask, are you sick? You seem to have aged 40 years."

His old pal responded, "Yes, I'm sick. I'm a sex addict."

Sex addiction will stress you out. It will age you, depress you, frustrate you, disappoint you, and abandon you in your darkest hour. Sex addiction will stress you out.

Fortunately, there is hope. Jesus said, "Come to me all who are stressed, and I will give you rest" (Matthew 11:28).

You need that rest. You need that Jesus.

Give your life to Jesus—the only one who can relieve your stress and give you peace.

Day 3
Boredom

You may be familiar with H.A.L.T. We tend to act out when we are hungry, angry, lonely, or tired. Add a "B" to the end. I know H.A.L.T.B. doesn't sound right, but it is.

B = Boredom

We act out when we are bored. We sometimes look at porn because we aren't looking at anything else. Many addicts attend some sort of intensive program for three days or even three months. But then they return to the "real world," only to find nothing back home has really changed. *They* have changed, but *their world* has not.

They have tools to use, books to read, and meetings to attend. But then it happens. Boredom. Down time. And this boredom becomes as much of a threat to their sobriety as a porn magazine sitting on the coffee table.

So what's the answer? Let me offer five very simple tips to avoid boredom.

1. New relationships
2. New hobbies
3. New habits
4. New books
5. New passion

The fact is, many of us get into trouble for one reason—we aren't getting into anything else. Part of your recovery plan is to stay occupied. Boredom is not your friend.

"Slothfulness casts into a deep sleep, and an idle person will suffer hunger" (Proverbs 19:15). Avoid boredom—at all costs.

Day 4
It's Not About Actions

Marcus Aurelius said, "The happiness of your life depends upon the quality of your thoughts; therefore, guard accordingly, and take care that you entertain no notions unsuitable to virtue and reasonable nature."

Thoughts lead to acts, which lead to habits, which lead to character, which leads to destiny. It all starts in the head.

Many addicts put too much stock in how they *act*, as opposed to how they *think*. Sobriety is not the absence of acting out; it is progressive victory over lust. And you can lust a thousand times a day and never act out again. But Jesus said that when we lust after someone, we have already crossed the line.

So what is the answer? It is found in one of Jesus' last teachings. "Watch and pray so that you will not fall into temptation. The spirit is willing, but the flesh is weak" (Matthew 26:41).

Whatever your triggers may be, the dual response is the same: watch and pray. First, be on the *watch* for temptations and intrusive thoughts. Second, when an image catches your eye or a fantasy invades your thoughts, do the "Double P"—*pop and pray*.

Marcus Aurelius had it right. "The happiness of your life depends upon the quality of your thoughts." Recovery does not begin with right actions; it ends there. The beginning of recovery is the next thought you choose to entertain.

Day 5
Toxic Relationships

In the account of the man we call the "rich young ruler," we find Jesus responding to a man of great wealth and influence, but who was not quite ready to go all in with his faith. Jesus let him walk away sad (Mark 10:22). In fact, we find about 25 passages in the New Testament that record Jesus walking away from someone.

What's the lesson? We need to learn when to exit toxic relationships.

Writing for *Psychology Today*, Dr. Asa Don Brown defined a toxic relationship as "any relationship that is unfavorable to you or others."

Chuck Swindoll was right when he said the main difference in our lives one year from now will be the people we spend time with.

Here's the bottom line. Healthy people hang with healthy people—a lot. To grow in your faith, maturity, and recovery, you need to connect with people who make you better by simply showing up. And you need to make some tough calls. Tough call #1—when to walk away. Jesus did it 25 times. Now it's your turn.

Think of one person in your life who only brings you down. You have done all you can for them. It's time to leave them in God's hands. It's time to walk away.

Day 6
What a Shame!

Shame is a bad thing—always. Guilt is okay, but never shame. Here's the difference. Guilt says what you have done is bad. Shame says *you* are bad. God would beg to differ.

Zephaniah 3:11 says, "On that day you, Jerusalem, will not be put to shame for the wrongs you have done to me."

If you are to overcome your past, you must first overcome your shame. Confess your sins to God, repent of them with a sincere heart, then let it go. You will never climb Mt. Recovery with the weight of shame draped around your shoulders. The burden is too heavy. Only One is strong enough to carry your shame, and he's already done it. That's why he said, "It is finished."

Dr. Jane Bolton writes, in *What We Get Wrong About Shame*, "When we are gripped by shame, we no longer think we have *done wrong*. We think we *are wrong*. We are somehow defective, inadequate, not good enough, not strong enough."

And that's when the enemy has us where he wants us. The problem is not shame, per se. The problem is what shame does to us. It cripples us with feelings of inadequacy. Shame tells those who will listen, "You don't *have* a problem; you *are* a problem!"

Jesus died for your shame. So let it go. Embrace the forgiveness of a God who created the second chance. The fact is, you can be victorious because you—in Christ—are good enough. You are strong enough.

Walk away from your shame and into the miracle of grace.

Day 7
The Test

Robert and James applied for the same job. They filled out the same test, and both got nine of ten questions correct. In fact, they even missed the same question. But after reviewing both tests, the company gave the job to Robert without hesitation.

James was outraged. He asked the boss, "Why did you give the job to Robert? We got the same score and even missed the very same question on the test."

The boss said, "Our decision was easy, James. On question #8, Robert answered, 'I don't know.' You answered, 'Neither do I.'"

In recovery, you have to do your own work. Even when you don't have the answer, and when you fail, the experience will serve you well in long-term recovery. You only fail the test if you quit before it is over.

Sobriety brings many tests. When you see an attractive person, you will be tested. When an invasive thought rushes to your mind, you will be tested. When you watch just about anything on television, you will be tested. And you can pass those tests, if you do your own work.

The Bible says, "My flesh and my heart may fail, but God is the strength of my heart and my portion forever" (Psalm 73:26).

In your fight for sobriety, you will be tested. And you may not win every battle or know the answer to every question. But you will grow through every test—if you do your own work.

Week 39
Outer Circle

"The closer we get to the outer circle, the more ground we will have to stay balanced."

- Siamrehab.com

THIS WEEK'S EXERCISE
Attend a New Meeting

Your outer circle activities are the things you do that contribute to your sobriety. These are areas where you need to strive for consistency, especially in the first year of your recovery. Here are some examples of typical outer circle activities:

- Prayer
- 12-Step work
- Family time
- Reading Scripture
- Meditation
- Recovery Day
- Church attendance
- Exercise
- Worship
- Therapy

Another outer circle activity is attending recovery meetings. It is possible to attend meetings and still not be sober. But it is nearly impossible to remain sober without attending meetings.

In Alcoholics Anonymous, there is an old expression that says, "There are three times when you should go to a meeting: when you don't feel like going, when you do feel like going, and at 8:00."

It is not a matter of how you feel. It is what you do that counts. Many, early in recovery, attend 90 meetings in 90 days. I found that to be very useful in my early recovery. These meetings provide insight, community, and encouragement. Your life may depend on attending meetings.

One of the things I have found most useful is to attend a new meeting every few weeks, either in my area or when I travel. This keeps my recovery from becoming stale and predictable.

Your first task is to find a "home meeting," one you are most committed to, if you have not done this already. You can find a local meeting easily. But for this week, your exercise is to attend a new meeting, or one you have not been to in at least three months. This can be a live meeting or a phone meeting. Here are a few websites that may help you find a meeting:

- Sexaholics Anonymous: sa.org
- Sex Addicts Anonymous: saa-recovery.org
- Celebrate Recovery: celebraterecovery.com
- Castimonia: castimonia.org
- 180 Recovery: 180recovery.com

Now, describe your feelings and experiences from this meeting, once you have attended, either in person or by phone. Try to identify at least one lesson you learned, which you can implement into your personal recovery plan.

The meeting I attended: _____

The date of the meeting: _____.

One lesson or principle I learned at this meeting: _____

_____

_____

Day 1
Patting Birds

Linus, of *Peanuts* fame, was taking a lot of heat because of his newly found "calling." He liked to pat birds on their heads. Distressed little birds would approach him, lower their feathered pates to be patted, sigh deeply, and then walk away satisfied. This brought Linus indescribable joy.

Charlie Brown and Lucy asked him why he was doing this.

"What's wrong with patting birds on their heads?" Linus asked.

"Are you kidding me?" Charlie Brown asked. "What's wrong with it is that nobody else is doing it!"

Most men struggle with porn. What sets the man in recovery apart from the crowd is that he's doing something about it. Most people you know have a problem. They need recovery on some level. But that requires much of us, so most people aren't doing it.

Joshua was willing to stand up for God even when no one else was doing it. "But if serving the Lord seems undesirable to you, then choose for yourselves this day whom you will serve . . . but as for me and my household, we will serve the Lord" (Joshua 24:15).

If you are going to overcome your addiction to sex and porn, you need to take the steps of recovery—even if nobody else is doing it.

Take the steps of recovery, whether anyone else does or not.

Day 2
Mack Robinson

In recovery, you cannot afford to fail. And the good news is that with God on your side, you don't have to.

The Scripture promises, "What then shall we say to these things? If God is for us, who can be against us?" (Romans 8:31).

History reminds us of the legendary Olympics of 1936. Among the four gold medals won by Jesse Owens was the one awarded for the 200-meter run on August 5. Owens set a new world record that day. But there is more to the story.

The world record that Owens set that day broke the "old" record, set just one day earlier by a 22-year-old runner named Mack Robinson. Like Owens, Robinson was a black American, running before an audience that included Adolf Hitler. Owens credited Robinson with making him better. "With Mack on my team, I knew I never had to run alone," he said.

Jesse Owens was better because Mack Robinson was on his team. And though you may have never heard of Mack Robinson, you may have heard of his younger brother, a baseball player named Jackie. Yes—Jackie Robinson.

In your race for sobriety, know this—you will never have to run alone.

Day 3
The Refuge of God

The words of the old hymn were written in Scotland in 1650.

"God is our refuge and our strength, our ever present aid.
And, therefore, though the earth remove, we will not be afraid.
The Lord of Hosts is on our side, our safety is secure;
The God of Jacob is for us, a refuge strong and sure."

Nahum 1:7 says, "The Lord is good, a strong refuge when trouble comes. He is close to those who trust him."

Recovery is a very difficult road to walk. Many abandon the journey out of fear, loneliness, or isolation. But when we feel deserted by others, we need to remember that we will never be deserted by God. He is for us, with us, and in us.

Writing *The True Christian Life*, John Calvin said, "Warned by such evidences of their spiritual illness, believers profit by their humiliations. Robbed of their foolish confidence in the flesh, they take refuge in the grace of God. And when they have done so, they experience the nearness of the divine protection which is to them a strong fortress."

I love Calvin's imagery. Addicts "profit by their humiliations" and "take refuge in the grace of God."

You have been humiliated by your addiction. But take heart. Better yet, take refuge—in the grace of the God who loves you still.

In the depths of your addiction, take refuge in God.

Day 4
Unplug

In trying to get well, we engage in many new activities: therapy, 12-Step work, disclosures, and more. But one of the best things we can do is to simply unplug.

The psalmist wrote, "I said, 'Oh, that I had the wings of a dove! I would fly away and be at rest'" (Psalm 55:6).

Novelist Anne Lamott said, "Almost everything will work again if you unplug it for a few minutes, including you."

Restlessness, anxiety, and stress are major contributors to addictions and poor health. The National Institute for Occupational Safety and Health (NIOSH) reports, "Health expenditures are nearly 50 percent greater for workers who report high levels of stress."

In recovery, we need to plug into the right things. But we also need to unplug. We need time to rest, to unwind, and to find God. And make no mistake—God can be found. But first we must unplug.

Learn to rest, to take a break, and simply unplug. The psalmist was right. You can fly like a dove. But first, you must find rest.

Day 5
Stay Close

It had been a great day. They were eye witnesses to the feeding of the 5,000. Now the disciples of Christ were riding high and they'd never look back, right? Wrong. We read, "That evening Jesus' disciples went down to the shore to wait for Jesus. But as darkness fell and Jesus still hadn't come back, they got into the boat and headed across the lake toward Capernaum. Soon a gale swept down upon them, and the sea grew very rough" (John 6:16-18).

We learn two lessons here. First, yesterday's victory is no guarantee of tomorrow's success. The disciples had just witnessed an amazing miracle. Surely, they'd stay on track now. But their newfound faith stayed with them for about two hours.

Second, it is important to wait on God. At the first sign of darkness and pending storms, the disciples left Jesus and went out on their own. They were willing to walk with him as long as they could do it on their own terms.

As a consequence, the disciples would have never made it to the other side of the lake, had Jesus not saved them—again. Henry Ford was right when he said, "Those who walk with God always reach their destination."

In recovery, life will be like that of the disciples. In the same day, they witnessed a great miracle and then encountered a harrowing storm. The key to survival is to never walk away from Christ.

When times are good, walk with Jesus. When times are bad, walk with Jesus. At all times—walk with Jesus.

Day 6
You Need Friends

Dr. Susan Whitbourne wrote a wonderful book on relationships titled *15 Reasons You Need Friends*. Her premise is simple. She writes, "You are a product of your friends."

Think about that—you are a product of your friends. Many of us have spent thousands of dollars on our education. Some commit countless hours to the gym. Others are meticulous about their diets. Many define themselves by their job, their income, or their house, car, or boat. They spend money they don't have to buy things they don't need to impress people they don't like.

But the real difference maker—in life and recovery—is friendships.

Chuck Swindoll likes to say, "There are two things that will determine the difference between where you are today and where you will be one year from now—the books you read and the people you spend time with."

Establishing friendships that will help you navigate successful recovery does not happen by accident. Real friendships are intentional.

The old prophet Amos asked, "Do two men walk together unless they have made an appointment?" (Amos 3:3).

You need to make an appointment with people who will feed your recovery. Pray for God to direct you to such people. You may find them at church, in a small group, or in a 12-Step meeting. Wherever you find them, find them! Why? Because you are the product of your friends.

Ask God to direct you to a few friends who will help feed your recovery.

Day 7
Holy God's

Every hour of every day, Christians all over the world sing the words of Chris Tomlin:

"We fall down, we lay our crowns—at the feet of Jesus. The greatness of mercy and love—at the feet of Jesus. And we cry holy, holy, holy. And we cry holy, holy, holy. And we cry holy, holy, holy is the Lamb."

God calls us to holiness. "Even before he made the world, God loved us and chose us in Christ to be holy and without fault in his eyes" (Ephesians 1:4).

Indeed, God's primary goal is to make us holy—that is, to form his character in us. Looking through the eyes of love, he already sees us as we will be when his work is done. Then he works out his goals for us in the arena of everyday life.

Holiness is the undesired pursuit of recovery. Rarely has a man sought holiness because it was fun, easy, or quickly rewarding. Spurgeon was right when he said, "Revenge, lust, ambition, pride, and self-will are too often exalted as the gods of man's idolatry; while holiness, peace, contentment, and humility are viewed as unworthy of a serious thought."

Holiness. It's time we started giving it serious thought.

If you wish to grasp this slippery thing we call sobriety, you must value the virtue of holiness above all else.

Week 40
20-Minute Miracle

"Count it all joy, my brothers, when you meet trials of various kinds,
for you know that the testing of your faith produces steadfastness.
And let steadfastness have its full effect, that you may be
perfect and complete, lacking in nothing."

- James 1:2-4

THIS WEEK'S EXERCISE
Practice the 20-Minute Miracle

One study estimated that the time span from when an addict feels a strong urge to act out and then actually does it is usually under ten minutes. We usually give in right away, or we stay strong. The exception is the man or woman whose primary acting out behavior involves paying for sex or meeting someone online. But even with them, the process begins quickly, as they go online or hop in their car to drive to a place where they should not go.

To those who feel like this urge is more than they can stand, I say three things.

1. What you feed, grows.

Sexual addiction is progressive. For example, if you masturbate today, you will likely be right back facing the same challenge tomorrow. And it only gets worse. There will be a time when what it took to satisfy your sexual appetite today is no longer enough.

2. Sex is not a need.

Someone once challenged me on this, insisting sex is a need. This was my response. I said, "I'm going to offer you four things. You can pick three of them for the next 30 days, but only three. You can have (a) food, (b) water, (c) oxygen, and/or (d) sex. Which one will you do without?" Here's the deal. You can't go 30 days without food, three days without water, or three minutes without oxygen. But you can go without sex. It is not a need.

3. If you can hold on for 20 minutes, you can hold on.

Within about 20 minutes after the dopamine rush, the urge will greatly diminish. You will no longer have the strong craving. If you can make it for 20 minutes, you can make it.

308

This 20-Minute Miracle has saved the sobriety of many of my clients. And it can be a huge tool in your toolbox, as well. But it is not enough to "white knuckle it" for 20 minutes. You need to distract your brain during this time. You need to refocus until the urge has diminished.

Below is a list of things you can do during these 20 minutes. Check the ones you will try. If, during this week, you find a need to practice this 20-Minute Principle, record your thoughts below.

20-Minute Checklist

_____ Pray

_____ Go for a walk

_____ Make a call

_____ Go for a drive

_____ Get with a nearby friend

_____ Read recovery material

_____ Cook a meal

_____ Read Scripture

_____ Engage in a hobby

_____ Go grocery shopping

_____ Quote Scripture

_____ Exercise

My reflections, having conducted this exercise: _____

_____

_____

_____

_____

_____

_____

_____

Day 1
Blame Yourself

You only have two options is life—blame others or accept responsibility. Consider the following advice.

Carol Burnett: "Only I can change my life. No one can do it for me." Willie Nelson: "You'll never get ahead by blaming your problems on other people." Oprah Winfrey: "You are responsible for your life. You can't keep blaming somebody else for your dysfunction. Life is really about moving on." George Bernard Shaw: "People are always blaming their circumstances for what they are. I don't believe in circumstances. The people who get on in this world are the people who get up and look for the circumstances they want, and if they can't find them, they make them."

The Apostle Paul: "Each one will have to bear his own load" (Galatians 6:5).

Yes, we are all products of our pasts. But we are only bound by those influences if we decide to live there—in the past. Let me suggest that no one but you can control the following:

1. Your attitude
2. Your words
3. Your actions

I repeat—you only have two options. You can blame others or you can accept responsibility. But if you want to get well, get going, and get ahead, you have only one option. You must accept responsibility for who you are, what you have done, and what will come next.

Regardless of how you got here, the journey to greatness begins with one step. And only one person will decide how you take that step. That person is you.

Day 2
Mind Games

Thomas Bailey Aldrich, the longtime editor of *The Atlantic Monthly*, commented, "A man is known by the company his mind keeps."

Let's talk about that.

Is it possible that we have placed too much emphasis on the things an addict does—including porn use, masturbation, and affairs? I say, yes.

Let me explain. It is what happens in a man's mind that dictates that man's actions. Before a man sleeps with a woman in his bed, he has already slept with her in his head—sometimes, dozens of times. No one ever looked at porn because they thought it was the sports section. They didn't go on a dating site looking to buy furniture.

The biggest sex organ is the brain. It is what a person does in his head that fuels the fires of addiction.

Solomon knew a little about multiple sex partners. And this is what he said: "As a man thinks in his heart, so is he" (Proverbs 23:7).

Thoughts precede actions. So make that your first priority—the company you keep—in your head.

Day 3
It's Not About What Happens to You

At the heart of every addiction you will find two things: trauma and isolation. And I have yet to meet the man or woman who said, "I asked for my trauma or isolation." But the good news is that the events of your past—and present/future—do not have to define you. There is one thing that matters far more than your circumstances.

How you react.

Dennis P. Kimbro said, "Life is ten percent what happens to us and ninety percent how we react to it."

The Bible promises us, "We are hard pressed on every side, but not crushed; perplexed, but not in despair; persecuted, but not abandoned; struck down, but not destroyed" (2 Corinthians 4:8-9).

You are a product of your past—good and bad. But it is what comes next that will define the rest of your life.

Try this. Identify something bad that has happened to you recently. It might be financial, relational, professional, or sexual. Now pray this: "God, grant me the serenity to accept the things I cannot change, the courage to change the things that I can, and the wisdom to know the difference."

Surrender it all to God—your past, your pain, and every circumstance that has come against you. Then, plan your next move, because it is your next move that matters most.

Day 4
The War Within

We often get this idea that the Apostle Paul had it all together, that he had risen above the common sins and temptations that derail the rest of us. Nothing could be further from the truth. Hear him in his own words:

"I know that good itself does not dwell in me, that is to say in my sinful nature. For I have the desire to do what is good, but I cannot carry it out" (Romans 7:18).

That is the war that rages within each of us. We want to do the right thing, but find ourselves coming up short. But I suggest that this struggle, of itself, is not a bad thing.

Frederick Douglass wrote, "Without a struggle there can be no progress."

So which side will win the battle? I suggest it is the side you feed the most. If you feed your addiction, expect a rough road ahead. But if you feed your recovery, expect success. And along the way, know that you will not likely win every battle.

Pope Paul VI said, "All life demands struggle."

Recovery may be the biggest struggle of all. But you only lose if you quit fighting. So stay in the fray, whether it feels like you are winning or not.

Engage the enemy today. Whatever the temptation, keep fighting. Feed your recovery with the things you know will work. Then keep at it. Eventually, freedom will be yours.

Day 5
The Step That Counts

I have observed the following pattern in acting out: (a) think it, (b) plan it, (c) do it, (d) hate it, (e) cover it, (f) do it again.

A client recently confided in me, "I spent hours thinking about how I would act out. I never intended to actually follow through with it. But the next thing I knew, there I was—in the midst of my old habit."

Marnie Ferree is right: "You can't stop at the acting out stage. You must interrupt the cycle before you get into your ritual."

I suggest that you forget about steps 3-6 in the pattern above. And don't even worry too much about step 1. The fact is, we all "think it" at some point. It's what we do with that invasive thought that matters. When we ritualize the thought by planning a way to act on it, we're dead in the water.

Dr. Caroline Leaf says, in *Switch On Your Brain*, "As we think, we change the physical nature of our brains. As we consciously direct our thinking, we can wire the toxic patterns of thinking and replace them with healthy thoughts."

The Bible simply says, "As a man thinks in his heart, so is he" (Proverbs 23:7).

The battle over addiction is won at Step 2—the planning stage. You must determine, starting today, that when the temptation hits, you will bounce your thoughts in a new direction.

Day 6
Baby Steps

Do you remember your first "baby steps"? Of course not. You have no memories from age one. Or do you?

The fact is, you can run now because you first learned to walk. And you learned to walk because you first learned how to take "baby steps." So, even though you no longer remember those first steps, they continue to pay dividends today.

The same is true in recovery. Take a few baby steps in your early recovery this week. Five years from now, you may not even remember taking these early steps. But they will prove vital to the journey you must start.

Rumi, a 13th-century Persian scholar, said it like this: "If all you can do is crawl, start crawling."

God wants you to experience freedom. He even promises you freedom: "Now the Lord is the Spirit, and where the Spirit of the Lord is, there is freedom" (2 Corinthians 3:17).

Freedom. Baby steps. You can't have one without the other.

Take baby steps today, so you can experience freedom tomorrow.

Day 7
Paramore

A congressman was asked about his attitude toward whiskey. He replied, "If you mean that demon drink that poisons the mind, pollutes the body, desecrates family life, and inflames sinners, I'm against it. But if you mean the elixir of Christmas cheer, the shield against winter chill, the taxable potion that puts needed funds into public coffers to comfort little crippled children, then I'm for it."

We can justify just about any behavior. But the truth is, the basis for most of our beliefs is self-indulgence. I vote for the candidate whose policies will help *me*. I obey the laws that benefit *me*. I pray prayers to bless *me*.

James 3:16 reads, "For where you have envy and selfish ambition, there you find disorder and every evil practice."

I've never heard the music of the modern rock band Paramore. But I love these lines from their hit song, *Playing God.*

"You don't deserve a point of view
If the only thing you see is you."

If you are to reach your maximum impact as a human being (and this includes sustained recovery), you have to embrace this truth—life is not all about you.

"You don't deserve a point of view if the only thing you see is you." That's not Scripture, but it is truth. So get outside yourself today, and do something to bless someone else.

Week 41
Solitude

"Solitude is painful when one is young, but delightful when one is more mature."

- Albert Einstein

THIS WEEK'S EXERCISE
Sit on It!

The Bible never says, "Be loud and know that I am God." We all know we need to be still before God, but most of us stink at the follow-through. Ours is a world that puts a premium on activity. We work hard, play hard, and party hard. The last thing we make time for is solitude.

We know that Jesus went into the mountain, Paul went into the wilderness, and Moses went into the dessert. But we are more comfortable going into the office, the bar, or the gym. We like noise.

A friend sent me a comic strip recently. It told of a man whose wife convinced him to turn off the TV for one night. The man discovered—for the first time—that when turned off, the TV screen becomes black.

Don't worry. I'm not going to ask you to go to a monastery for a week. We'll start small. Give solitude a try for just 15 minutes.

Here's what you will do—*nothing.*

Am I going too fast for you? For 15 minutes, you will not watch anything, read anything, or say anything. You won't even pray, unless you consider silence a form a prayer. (It is.)

Plan a time and pick a place where you can sit and do nothing. It is important that this place be outside, where you can best experience the world as it was before God made big buildings and fast cars.

During these 15 minutes, simply enjoy the presence of God. Use all of the senses that he gave you. Afterward, jot down what you heard, saw, felt, smelled, and tasted of God and his presence.

Date of exercise: _____

Place of exercise: _____

How you experienced God and his presence:

What you heard: _____

What you saw: _____

What you felt: _____

What you smelled: _____

What you tasted: _____

Summary: _____

_____

_____

_____

Day 1
The 4-Letter Word of Recovery

There is a four-letter word for recovery. *Rest*. It is not an option. It's in the Ten Commandments. "You have six days in your week to work, but the seventh day is a day of rest" (Exodus 20:9).

Why is rest important to our recovery? Because it offers a break from stress, and stress triggers addiction. There's an old acronym in recovery we call "H.A.L.T." We tend to act out when we are *hungry*, *angry*, *lonely*, or *tired*.

The National Sleep Foundation says we need seven to nine hours of sleep every day. The National Institute for Occupational Safety and Health has found 12 benefits to a day of rest. The first is that it reduces stress. And nothing triggers addiction like stress.

I suggest you go a step further. Some of the best advice my sponsor ever gave me was to have a Recovery Day every month or so. A Recovery Day is a day of rest. It includes solitude, reading recovery material, meditation, and prayer.

William Wadsworth wrote, "Rest and be thankful." Embrace rest. It's God's four-letter word for recovery. Every seven days you need a day of rest. Your recovery depends on it.

Day 2
The Wise Men

Wise men still seek Jesus.

Let's review the story of the wise men, as told in Matthew, chapter 2. We learn three principles from their story that apply to recovery.

1. They were in tune with their Higher Power. They came a great distance in search of the child Jesus. "We have come to worship him" (Matthew 2:2). Their search took them to King Herod and involved following a star. They were relentless in their search. The same is true of recovery. You will not find it apart from a relentless pursuit of your Higher Power.

2. They offered great sacrifices. "They opened their treasures and presented him with gifts of gold, and of incense, and of myrrh" (2:11). These gifts carried great meaning, sacrifice, and value. Likewise, recovery will cost you something, or it

won't stick. Like the wise men, in order to gain something, you must give something up.

3. They went home a different way. "They returned to their country by another route" (2:12). When we encounter Jesus, we live differently from who we were before we came. The same is true of recovery. We have a "come as you are" Savior, but he is not a "stay as you were" Lord. True recovery starts with an encounter with our Higher Power and results in change.

Wise men still seek Jesus. And they bring him the gift of sacrifice. What gift will you give him today?

My old pastor taught me this poem by Christina Rossetti. I suggest you embrace it today, that recovery may be yours for a lifetime. *"What can I give him, small as I am? If I were a shepherd, I'd give him a lamb. If I were a wise man, I'd surely do my part. But what can I give him? I can give him my heart."*

Day 3
Lift Your Eyes

The only route to a certain harbor in Italy leads through a narrow channel between dangerous rocks and shoals. Over the years many ships have crashed as crews have tried to navigate through the channel. To solve this problem authorities mounted three lights on three huge poles in the harbor to guide ships safely into port. When a ship's captain lines up the three lights and all three appear as one light, the ship can proceed safely up the narrow channel. Everything depends on the captain's eyes. If he sees two or three lights he knows he's off course and in danger.

In the same way, the songwriter of Psalm 123 turned his eyes toward God. "I lift my eyes to you, to you who sit enthroned in heaven" (Psalm 123:1).

Guillaume de Saluste du Barta wrote, "The world is a stage where God's omnipotence, justice, knowledge, love, and providence do act the parts."

Everything in creation screams: "Look to God!" As you navigate the narrow channel of recovery, nothing is more important than lining up your focus. It is only when you lift your eyes to God that you can safely reach your intended destination.

Lift your eyes to God today. When the channel is narrow and the waters are choppy, that will be the only way you can stay on course.

Day 4
The Divorce of Marilyn Monroe

On January 21, 1962, Marilyn Monroe asked Judge Miguel Gomez for a plate of tacos and enchiladas. Then she filed for divorce from Arthur Miller, her third husband. One year later, she took her own life.

Born Norma Jean Mortenson, the "blonde bombshell" was a sex symbol, star of 24 movies, and had a wealth of $10 million at the time of her death at age 36. She had been married to Joe DiMaggio and had romantic ties to Marlon Brando and President John F. Kennedy. Monroe had fame and fortune. What she didn't have was peace.

At the height of her popularity, Monroe said, "I am trying to find myself. Sometimes, that's not easy." In another interview, the star admitted, "Dreaming about being an actress is more exciting than being one."

What do you dream about? If, like Marilyn Monroe, you are chasing pleasure, prepare to be disappointed. Solomon, talking to himself, concluded, "I said to myself, 'Come now, I will test you with pleasure to find out what is good.' But that also proved to be meaningless" (Ecclesiastes 2:1).

I asked a fellow sex addict, "Why do you act out?" He said, "That's simple. It brings me pleasure."

The problem is, pleasure only satisfies for the moment.

If, like Marilyn Monroe, you are trying to find yourself through pleasure, let me suggest this—find God first.

Day 5
Awareness

I have a dear friend who recently lost his wife of 60 years. He poured himself into his work, where he has served as the senior pastor of a church that he planted in 1966. He turned to family and friends for comfort. But the pain just wouldn't go away. And then he began to pray this prayer: "May my awareness of your presence be greater than my awareness of my wife's absence."

If you have lost your husband or wife to sex addiction, perhaps this would be a good prayer for you to embrace: "May my awareness of your presence be greater than my awareness of the loss of my spouse to his addiction."

The answer to a broken marriage is not a new marriage. The answer is a personal, intimate relationship with your God. Nothing less will suffice.

The Bible promises, "The Lord is good to those whose hope is in him, to the one who seeks him" (Lamentations 3:25).

The pain of betrayal and loss cannot be overstated. Will you always be aware of the loss of this person you loved and trusted with your whole heart? Of course, you will. The key is not to forget your loss, but to remember your God.

Pray it with me: "May my awareness of your presence be greater than my awareness of the loss of my spouse to his addiction."

Day 6
The 7ᵗʰ Step

Confucius said, "Humility is the solid foundation of all virtues."

The Twelve Steps and Twelve Traditions says this: "The attainment of greater humility is the foundational principle of each of AA's twelve steps."

The Seventh Step is a perfect opportunity to embrace humility. You can't work this Step without it.

In this critical Step, we "humbly ask him to remove all our shortcomings." In previous Steps, we identify our shortcomings; in Step 7, we take action. It is not enough to list our character defects, or to share them with others. Nor is it enough to try to overcome them. Recovery is a spiritual program. We must engage God in every Step. We must ask him to do for us what we could not do for ourselves. And this demands humility.

One of the purest ways to work the Seventh Step is to pray the Seventh Step Prayer, which I try to do three times a day:

"My Creator, I am now willing that you should have all of me, good and bad. I pray that you now remove from me every single defect of character which stands in the way of my usefulness to you and to my fellows. Grant me strength as I go out from here to do your bidding."

Day 7
I Feel Shame—Is That Good?

Do you feel shame for what you've done? I suggest that is never good, and it is not from God. Let me explain.

There is a difference between guilt and shame. Guilt says, "I've done a bad thing." Shame says, "I am a bad person." Guilt can be a good thing, as it can be the tool of the Holy Spirit to redirect our paths. But when we live in shame, we define ourselves by our actions. Psychologist Joseph Burgo says it like this: "Shame reflects psychological damage that impedes growth."

Dr. Brene Brown goes even further: "Shame is a destructive force, especially for those who suffer from addictions." And Dr. Gabor Mate says that "shame furthers addiction and can have fatal consequences."

We all have guilt, for all have sinned (Romans 3:23). But "there is no condemnation for those who are in Christ Jesus" (Romans 8:1).

If you are still living in your addiction, you are guilty. You are living apart from the plan of God. That rush of remorse you feel every time you relapse is God's way of prodding you toward repentance. But God is not the author of shame. Let me say it like this: there is nothing you can ever do that will make God love you more, and there is nothing you have ever done that has made God love you less.

If you are a follower of Christ, claim his forgiveness and grace. When you fail, embrace the guilt that the Holy Spirit proclaims over your life. Repent. Then move on. Live in freedom. To do less is to deny the grace of God. And that would be a shame.

Week 42
Housecleaning

*"I hate housework. You make the beds, you wash
the dishes, and six months later you have
to start all over again."*

- Joan Rivers

THIS WEEK'S EXERCISE
Clean House

We have some dear friends who have a home in our city of Bradenton, Florida. But this is not their primary residence. When they are not here, we sometimes go by the house for them, to make sure everything is working. We check the lightbulbs, faucets, toilets, etc. And when someone has been staying at the house, we take out the trash.

In most neighborhoods, "regular" trash is picked up a couple of days a week. Recycled trash is picked up on another day. But in order for the trash guys to pick it up, we have to haul it to the curb. They won't walk through your front door and rummage through your house looking for your trash. That would be creepy.

You may want them to take your trash away, as far as the east is from the west—to never be seen again. But until you make the effort to haul it to the curb, your trash isn't going anywhere. And the longer you hang onto it, the more it will stink.

In recovery, you need to clean house from time to time. You need to take out your "trash." This trash comes in many forms:

- Old letters
- Old pictures
- Old devices
- Old magazines
- Old web links
- Hidden cash
- Hidden phone numbers
- Hidden email addresses

In a sense, you need to destroy your old trash. But what you really need to do—on a spiritual level—is to take your trash to the curb. Let God destroy it. Yes, you need to get rid of the materials you are holding onto. But you also need to confess your trash to God in prayer, with a repentant heart. Let's get started.

Getting rid of the physical evidence:

- _____
- _____
- _____
- _____
- _____

Confessing the hidden "trash" of your heart:

- _____
- _____
- _____
- _____
- _____

Day 1
Taking Out the Garbage

John Piper tells the story about the time he had a fight with his wife early in their marriage. He needed a break from the argument, so he left the house to take the garbage down the street to the pick-up spot. He says, "As I walked down the driveway toward the street where we set the garbage, the sun broke through the morning clouds. To this day, the profoundness of that moment grips me. Here I was huffing and puffing with my hurt feelings and desires for vindication, and God, who had every right to strike me dead, opened the window of heaven and covered me with pleasure. I recall stopping and letting it soak in. It felt like paradise—garbage in hand."

The Bible says, "The heavens declare the glory of God; the skies proclaim the work of his hands . . . In the heavens God has pitched a tent for the sun" (Psalm 19:1, 4).

What was true for John Piper is also true for you and me. We all have garbage we need to take out. We need to take it to the cross, God's pick-up spot. That's where we lay our garbage down.

There is an interesting promise for those of us willing to release our garbage. We experience God's glory and his redeeming grace in the process. God does not wait until we are garbage-free to reveal his glory. He has "pitched a tent" of blessing for each of us who are in the process of taking out the garbage.

What garbage have you been hanging onto? It's time to let it go. Then prepare for the blessing in the journey, not just the destination.

We all have garbage to take out. Start bagging it up today, then take it to the cross. And prepare to meet God along the way.

Day 2
Riding Vacuum Cleaners

Housecleaning is not fun, but it is necessary.

Roseanne Barr said, "I'm not going to vacuum until Sears makes one you can ride on."

Housecleaning is not fun, but it is necessary.

Recovery is all about cleaning house. The Bible says, "Be diligent to be found by him without blot or blemish" (2 Peter 3:14). As followers of Christ, we are to make every effort to live spotless lives. But that is impossible until we learn to spot the spots. And that's where the Holy Spirit comes in. He stands ready to point out every spot that needs removing.

Housecleaning is not fun, but it is necessary.

The process of cleaning house can start today. Invite the Holy Spirit to reveal to you those character defects that are getting in the way of full recovery. Ask him to spot the spots you cannot spot so you can remove those spots. Why?

Housecleaning is not fun, but it is necessary.

You may have taken out the trash—ridding your life of porn, secret cash, and improper images on social media. But there are still some areas you need to clean up. And that process can begin today.

Day 3
Clean Glasses

On the road to recovery, it is important that we do a bit of introspection from time to time. David prayed, "Search me, God, and know my heart; test me and know my concerns. See if there is any offensive way in me; lead me in the everlasting way" (Psalm 139:23-24).

Seth Haines spoke for too many of us in *Coming Clean: A Story of Faith*. In his own transparency, he admitted, "I've become dependent upon something other than the God I claim."

Total, absolute dependency on God is essential to lasting sobriety. A huge sign of God's work in your life is that you can honestly pray, "Search me, God, and know my heart." It is when you welcome the spotlight of the Holy Spirit upon your life that you are ready to move forward in your recovery.

Every problem has a solution. For the addict, that solution is coming clean, admitting that we don't have it all together and that we don't always see life with clear eyes. As British dramatist Aaron Hill said, "Don't call the world dirty just because you forgot to clean your glasses."

It's time to clean your glasses. Seek God today—with all your heart. Ask him to open your eyes to anything in your life that needs his caring attention. Hold nothing back.

Pray this right now—"Search me, God, and know my heart; test me and know my concerns. See if there is any offensive way in me; lead me in the everlasting way."

Day 4
Dirty Laundry

A lady noticed that her neighbors were hanging their laundry out to dry on a line in their back yard. She reported to her husband over several weeks, "Every time our neighbors hang their laundry to dry, I notice their clothes still look dirty. They must not be able to afford laundry detergent."

After a few months, the lady was excited as she told her husband, "Our neighbors finally cleaned their clothes! Their laundry is hanging on the line in their backyard, like always. But everything looks so clean now!"

Her husband laughed as he told her, "Their laundry isn't any cleaner. The difference is that I cleaned our windows!"

We all view the world through dirty glass. Paul said we would never see things clearly in this life (1 Corinthians 13:12).

You can spend your life critiquing the shortcoming of your husband, wife, or some other child of God. But you have enough of your own dirty laundry to keep you occupied for a while. So if you want to clean up the world, start there.

Your job is not to inspect other people's dirty laundry, but to take care of your own. Take all the time you need to become completely Christlike. Then, if you have any time left over (you won't), go fix someone else.

Day 5
Cleaning House

We used to have a Cocker Spaniel named Duffy. She was one happy mess. Her bladder was unable to control her joy. We were always cleaning up after her. She slobbered horribly. When she'd run or shake her head, slobber went everywhere. What she messed up, we cleaned up.

One day, due to a back problem that is common among Cockers, Duffy became paralyzed. She couldn't walk or get to her food dish. We spent a king's ransom on her back surgery, knowing it may not be successful. Then we had to just wait and see. We fed her by hand and carried her outside where she could at least enjoy the view.

It took a few weeks, but eventually, she began to move again and she fully recovered. But she was still a mess. So why did we continue to clean up after her, no matter how bad it got? It's simple. We loved our dog more than we hated her mess.

You are a mess. But know this. God loves you more than he hates your mess.

We have this guarantee from God: "Their sins and lawless acts will I remember no more" (Hebrews 10:17). That's a pretty amazing promise.

God is in the housecleaning business. What we mess up, he cleans up. Then it's our turn to respond.

A.W. Tozer said, "You have been forgiven, so act like it!"

You have made a mess, but God has cleaned house. Now you are forgiven—so act like it!

Live like a child of the King. And if you ever make a mess of things again, remember this—God loves you more than he hates your mess.

Day 6
Why Addicts Lie

Here's some shocking news, hot off the press. *Addicts lie.* Okay, take a minute to catch your breath. It's true—addicts lie. But let's dig a little deeper. Let me suggest seven reasons addicts lie, adapted from an article by Dr. David Sack titled *7 Honest Reasons Addicts Lie.*

1. To preserve their addiction. If the addict acknowledges the gravity of his addiction, he can no longer justify his lifestyle.
2. To avoid reality. To preserve his sanity, the addict constructs an alternate reality in which he must conclude he doesn't really have a problem.
3. To avoid confrontation. Loved ones rarely sit idly by as the addict self-destructs. So he must cover up with a dishonest appearance of sobriety at all costs.
4. Out of denial. Even in the face of overwhelming evidence, the addict lies in order to convince himself he doesn't really have a problem.
5. They think they're different. The addict convinces himself that, unlike others, he can stop anytime.
6. Out of shame. The addict fears that if he is truly known, he won't be fully loved.
7. Because they can. Loved ones have turned a blind eye long enough that the addict can "get away" with his double life.

Yep, addicts lie. And they're good at it. You can still trust them—if you are willing to listen to their behaviors and not their words.

"Let him who lies, lie no more" (Ephesians 4:25).

Day 7
One Step

Every journey begins with the first step.

Small steps lead to a great destiny. Addition comes before multiplication, crawling before walking, and high school before college.

You have doubtlessly heard the following question. How do you eat an elephant? Of course the answer is, one bite at a time. (Perhaps a greater question would be this: Why do you want to eat an elephant?)

Let's apply this principle to recovery. It boils down to this—always. *Do the next best thing.*

An old Chinese proverb says, "Be not afraid of growing slowly; be afraid only of standing still."

In your recovery, you don't need to take big steps. In fact, I don't believe big steps are even possible. All recovery is taken one small step at a time—going to meetings, saying the Serenity Prayer, attending a therapy session. For others, this small step may be getting on Covenant Eyes, joining an accountability group, or getting a 12-Step sponsor.

Every journey begins with the first step. And it continues with the next step, and then the next step after that.

Take one step in recovery today. And remember, no step in the right direction is a step too small.

Week 43
Confession

"Sacrifice, discipline, and prayer are essential. We gain strength through God's Word. And when we fumble due to sin – and it's gonna happen – confession puts us back on the field."

- Lou Holtz

THIS WEEK'S EXERCISE
Write a Deathbed Confession

Are you ready for a morbid exercise? Well, we have one for you! First, the background.

Confession is good for the soul. King David said it like this: "I gave an account of my ways and you answered me" (Psalm 119:26). David knew what many of us have yet to understand—God can only heal what we reveal.

Is there anything you are still holding onto? Is there anything you have yet to get out, to confess to God and another human being? No one will see this exercise, unless you choose to share it with them. This is only meant to be between you and God.

If you were on your deathbed, I'm guessing you would want to make sure everything was right between you and God. You wouldn't want there to be any unconfessed sin. So this is your chance. Write a deathbed confession to God—telling him anything you have been holding onto.

My Deathbed Confession

Dear God, _____

_____

_____

_____

_____

_____

_____

_____

_____

Day 1
The Tell-Tale Heart

Edgar Allan Poe's short story, *The Tell-Tale Heart*, tells the gruesome story of a murderer who hides his victim's body under the floorboards of his house. He is so confident that he cannot be discovered that he invites police investigators into his house, where he cheerfully answers all of their questions, while standing just above the corpse.

Then the murderer hears the sound of a beating heart from below his feet. He wonders why the police don't seem to hear it, as the beating gets louder. Though the officers know nothing, the man finally loses it and confesses his crime.

Geoffrey Chaucer said, "The guilty think all talk is of themselves." In other words, the guilty become consumed in the destitution of their souls.

The Bible says, "Whoever conceals his sins does not prosper, but the one who confesses and renounces them finds mercy" (Proverbs 28:13).

John Adams said, "Great is the guilt of an unnecessary war."

One of the most unnecessary wars is the one that rages in the heart of a man who has something to hide. A man is crippled by his guilt and buried by his secrets. The key to recovery is not living a sin-free life. It is outing our mistakes before they destroy us.

Day 2
The Key to the Key

The key to a fresh start is forgiveness. And the key to forgiveness is confession. Bruce Lee said it like this: "Mistakes are always forgivable, if one has the courage to admit them."

One day, children were lined up in the cafeteria of a Christian school, waiting to buy lunch. At the end of the line was a large pile of apples. Someone had written a note and placed it by the apples. It read, "Take only one. God is watching."

Beyond the apples was a small table with three plates of chocolate chip cookies. One of the boys wrote his own note and placed it by the cookies. It read, "Take all you want. God is watching the apples."

That's how a lot of us do life. We do what we think we can get away with. But in recovery, we must come clean. We need the forgiveness that only God can supply. But that only comes when we admit our mistakes.

Those who confess their sins to God have this promise. "God does not punish us for all our sins; he does not deal harshly with us, as we deserve. For his unfailing love toward those who fear him is as great as the height of the heavens above the earth. He has removed our sins as far from us as the east is from the west" (Psalm 103:10-12).

The same God who is watching the apples is watching you. And he sees your mistakes. But when you confess them to him, He will see them no more.

Day 3
The Hardest Nine Words You'll Ever Say

It didn't come out of my mouth easily. In fact, I attended dozens of counseling sessions and a half dozen 12-Step meetings before I could bring myself to say it. The words came from a trembling basket of emotion.

"My name is Mark and I'm a sex addict."

And that's when the healing began.

Nothing is more difficult for a Type-A personality than saying, "I'm wrong. I have a problem and I can't solve it myself."

I knew I had a problem for years before anyone else did. Like most of us, I struggled with my conscience, trying to make peace within my heart. I lived in denial of what I had done and who I was. I minimized it. I worked hard to "be good," treated others well, served God, and gave a tenth of my income to the church. I read my Bible and prayed daily. But still, I had this problem.

I was born with a built-in alarm clock that went off every time I had a relapse. It was God's way of holding me accountable. It was his way of breathing Romans 2:15 into my heart all over again: "Their own conscience and thoughts either accuse them or tell them they are doing right."

Recovery can only come when we admit that our issues actually run a lot deeper than right vs. wrong. Carl Jung said, "The pendulum of the mind alternates between sense and nonsense, not between right and wrong."

Like the prodigal, I had to come to my senses and admit it. "I am a sex addict."

Day 4
I Confess

The first step to recovery is to recognize you have a problem—and not minimize it.

On the hit show, *Beverly Hills 90210*, Brandon Walsh, played by Jason Priestly, said, "You can't be a little addicted."

It's time to confess your struggle to the one who can do something about it. David said, "The one who confesses and renounces his sin finds mercy" (Psalm 28:13).

Kristen Wetherell, writing for The Gospel Coalition, said it like this: "Confession and repentance are an integral part of making progress in the Christian life."

Behind every recovery story is a time when the addict said to God, "I have a problem. I cannot beat this thing in my own power. I confess my sin, my struggle, my addiction. And I turn to you, begging for your forgiveness and cleansing. I turn my life over to you and your care."

Confess your addiction to the One who has the power to do something about it. Admit your shortcomings, your failed attempts to get well. Reach out to him. Get on your knees, pray, repent, and confess your absolute reliance on God. Will this bring an end to your problems? No—but it will bring a beginning to your recovery.

Day 5
Coming Clean

The question is not whether you will make mistakes and say things that are hurtful in the future. It's a matter of when and to what degree—and what you do next. Legendary coach Lou Holtz said, "When we fumble due to a sin—and it's gonna happen—confession puts us back on the field."

When you have a slip or relapse, or just say an unkind word, you need to own it and come clean. True confession is void of any minimizing, excuse-making, rationalizing, or blame-shifting.

The Bible says it very directly: "Tell the Israelites: When a man or woman commits a sin against another, that person acts unfaithfully toward the Lord and is guilty. The person is to confess the sin he has committed. He is to pay full compensation, add a fifth of its value to it, and give it to the individual he has wronged" (Number 5:6-7).

The David Crowder Band captured the essence of coming clean with their hit song, *Forgiven*. Some of the lyrics: "I'm the one who held the nail. It was cold between my fingertips. I've hidden in the garden. I've denied You with my very lips."

Another line: "I've done things I wish I hadn't done. I've seen things I wish I hadn't seen. Just the thought of Your amazing grace. And I cry, 'Jesus, forgive me!'"

You and I may never meet this side of heaven. But I know two things about you. First, you have made mistakes. Second, it's time to come clean.

Day 6
I Beg Your Pardon

In the opening of Paul's letter to the Ephesian church, he listed our blessings in Christ. One of those blessings is forgiveness. Paul wrote, "In him we have redemption through his blood, the forgiveness of our trespasses, according to the riches of his grace" (Ephesians 1:7).

In his commentary on Ephesians, John MacArthur wrote, "Forgiveness is the soil in which blessings are cultivated."

Henry Ward Beecher spoke of God's forgiveness. "God pardons like a mother, who kisses the offense into everlasting forgiveness."

Many people have something in their pasts that they can't quite shake—not just thoughtless mistakes, but deliberate, foolish choices. Like a ghost, each memory haunts them. This leads to regret. They wonder, "Can God really forgive me?"

From heaven's rafters, the answer is deafening: "YES!" God can and will. He is in the forgiveness business. If you have come up short in your battle for purity, if you have suffered a slip or relapse, take it to God with a sincere heart. Beg his pardon. He stands ready to forgive.

Day 7
Deathbed Confessions

Have you ever heard a deathbed confession? God has heard millions of them. So let's do a fun little exercise. If you could look ahead to age 80 or 90 and imagine yourself laying on what would become your deathbed, and if you were to confess one final thing to God, what would it be?

The man on the cross next to Jesus nailed it: "Lord, remember me when you come into your kingdom" (Luke 23:42).

Perhaps you aren't even that big on prayer. But there's something about knocking on death's door that makes a person want to hear a voice from the other side.

Dolly Parton said, "You don't see too many atheists on the deathbed. They all start cramming then."

Here's my suggestion—don't wait to cram. I've done that—for just about every test I ever took in college. Here's what I learned. If you wait to cram for the test at the last hour, you might pass the test, but you won't do as well as the guy who prepared well in advance.

I suggest you get your confessions out of the way now. Confess your struggles and addictions. Get it all out. That way, when the final exam is given, you'll be ready.

Week 44
Money

*"Money is only something you need
in case you don't die tomorrow."*

- Wall Street

THIS WEEK'S EXERCISE
Follow the Money

Being accountable for their finances has saved many sex addicts from acting out and losing their freedom and family. The following techniques can stop several forms of acting out instantly. For many, most acting out behaviors require money. Money is what makes the sick, illicit sexual world go around. Without money, even in the addict's lost desperate emotional state, he cannot purchase anything. Accountability and money can save your sobriety.

How this can be practiced is a very individual matter. Below, you will read some methods for financial accountability that you should find very helpful. These are practices you can start this week, and then carry forward. Typically, it takes six to twelve months to establish enough sobriety to begin to loosen some of these parameters.

Check the specific strategies you will engage, starting this week:

_____ Limit credit card use and show statements to your spouse.

_____ Use checks instead of credit cards and review your bank statement with your spouse.

_____ Eliminate any separate bank accounts.

_____ Carry a limited amount of cash, perhaps under $20.

_____ Do not hide any cash.

_____ Keep receipts for all expenditures.

_____ Review any spending with your spouse at the end of each day.

_____ Other: _____

_____ Other: _____

_____ Other: _____

Day 1
Money Trap

I learned something from my 30 years as a senior pastor. People act funny when you talk about money. But money matters—a lot. John Wesley said, "Make all you can, save all you can, and give all you can." Woody Allen mused, "Money is better than poverty, if only for financial reasons." And Jerry Seinfeld observed, "Dogs have no money. Isn't that amazing? They're broke their entire lives, but that never steals their joy."

Money—or lack thereof—steals a lot of joy.

What does this have to do with addiction? Dr. Elizabeth Hartley explains, "Financial problems are often a symptom of behavioral addictions."

I can relate to the man who lamented, "I'm so poor, there's a kid in India with my picture on his refrigerator."

But it's true. What you do with your money says a lot. That's why Paul warned, "Those who want to be rich fall into temptation, a trap, and many foolish and harmful desires, which plunge people into ruin and destruction. For the love of money is a root of all kinds of evil, and by craving it, some have wandered away from the faith and pierced themselves with many griefs" (1 Timothy 6:9-10).

Having money is not sinful. Many heroes of the Bible had money: Abraham, Jacob, Job, David, Solomon, Lydia, Joseph of Arimathea. And that's okay; the problem is when money has you. So learn to enjoy money—but don't crave it, for that is a sign of addiction.

Day 2
The Acceptable Addiction

Angela Kelly won $72 million in Britain's biggest lottery. Within a few years, she lost most of her friends, gained a lot of weight, and became a recluse. She called the lotto win "the worst day of my life." Mike Tyson won $300 million as a boxer. He filed for bankruptcy in 2003. And Burt Reynolds filed for bankruptcy in 1996 with over $10 million in debt.

Money—it's the acceptable addiction. Very few people have just one addiction. For many addicts, money is a companion to their other substance or behavioral addictions.

We know the Scripture that says, "Do not fix your hope on the uncertainty of riches" (1 Timothy 6:17). Still, it is a struggle.

Dr. John Moore, Editor-in-Chief of Guy Counseling, identifies five signs that you may have an addiction to money:

1. Your thoughts are consumed with making money.
2. You practice risky behaviors.
3. Your self-worth is tied to cash.
4. You don't spend on yourself.
5. You isolate and obsess.

Fortunately, there is a way out: "Lay up for yourselves treasures in heaven" (Matthew 6:20).

Day 3
Show Me the Money!

One of the biggest movies of 1996 was *Jerry Maguire*, starring Tom Cruise. Maguire managed the football career of Ron Tidwell, played by Cuba Gooding, Jr. Tidwell was Maguire's last client, and he didn't want to lose him. On a phone call, Maguire asked Tidwell what he needed to do to keep him, and the player replied, "We have a personal family motto, Jerry. It's very simple. Show me the money."

That's a good line for the wife of a sex addict. "Show me the money." Addicts spend a lot of money on their habits. Porn is a $16.9 billion industry in the United States.

Addicts hide two things—their habit and their money. Each year, the average American spends $209 on lotto tickets, $251 on beer, and $51 on porn. But try this. Sometime today, walk up to an average American and ask him, "Last year, did you spend $209 on lotto tickets, $251 on beer, and $51 on porn?" I'm guessing he'll deny it.

More specifically, sex addicts hide their money from their spouses. If you are married to someone with an addiction, know this—the way he handles his money will tell the story. If he is willing to be real and seek recovery, he won't mind the big question.

"Show me the money."

Day 4
It's All About Money

Oscar Wilde, Irish playwright, wrote in *The Picture of Dorian Gray*, "Young people imagine that money is everything, and when they grow older, they know it is."

Boxing legend Joe Lewis admitted, "I don't like money, actually. But it quiets my nerves."

Speaking on the needs of a woman, Sophie Tucker, early 20th century entertainer, said, "From birth to 18 a girl needs good parents; from 18 to 35 she needs good looks; from 35 to 55 she needs a good personality, and from 55 on she needs cash."

Money is good, but it has limitations. It can buy medicine, but not health; a house, but not a home; companionship, but not friends; entertainment, but not happiness; food, but not an appetite; a bed, but not sleep; a crucifix, but not a Savior; a good life, but not an eternal life.

The Bible says, "He who loves money never has enough" (Ecclesiastes 5:10). The same is true for everything money can buy—including sex. Here's the thing about sex—it is a desire, not a need. (Intimacy is a need.) I've known guys who have spent as much as $250,000 on sex. But it was never enough.

We need to quit expecting money and the things it can buy to do for us what only God can do.

Day 5
Emancipation

It is listed in legislative history as "Proclamation 95." It was an executive order that changed the lives of 3.5 million Americans in a single day. That day was January 1, 1863. The executive order is better remembered as the Emancipation Proclamation. And with that order, President Lincoln freed every slave who lived in the South. But they could not realize that freedom as long as the Civil War continued—unless they found their way to the North.

Jesus has declared your freedom. That's what "It is finished" was all about. But you still have to do the work of recovery to find the Promised Land.

Scripture tells us that "people are slaves to whatever has mastered them" (2 Peter 2:19).

If you want to know who or what has mastered you, I suggest you look in two places: your calendar and your checkbook. It is where we spend our time and money that becomes our master.

But God has a better way. John MacArthur said it simply: "To be a Christian is to be a slave of Christ."

The fact is, you are a slave to something. If you spend an inordinate amount of time and money on sex, that is your master. The good news is that you have been emancipated. Now it's time to do the work necessary to fully enjoy the blessing of that glorious freedom.

Day 6
For the Love of Money

There's an old saying that describes the spending habits of most Americans. We spend money we don't have on things we don't need to impress people we don't like.

In the movie *Wall Street*, Gordon Gekko, played by Michael Douglas, spoke for so many of us. "What's worth doing is worth doing for money."

Americans have a convoluted view of the relationship between money and happiness. As a nation, we owe $793 billion in credit card debt, have only $400 per family in savings, but still spend $70 billion on the lottery.

The time and money spent on porn is even more alarming. Every second, there are 28,000 viewers spending a total of $3,000 on Internet porn. The average American viewed 221 pages of Internet porn in 2015, and porn is an $11 billion industry.

And it gets worse every year, because porn—like money—never satisfies. Just ask the man who had the most money—and women—in the world. Solomon said, "Whoever loves money never has enough" (Ecclesiastes 5:10).

It's time to get off the crazy train. Quit chasing money and the things money can buy—because it never satisfies. As we say in 12-Step meetings, "There is one who has all power—that one is God. May you find him now!"

Day 7
What Gives?

John Bunyan said, "You have not lived today until you have done something for someone who can never repay you."

C.S. Lewis wrote, "The proper aim of giving is to put the recipients in a state where they no longer need your gifts."

Better yet, Jesus famously said, "It is more blessed to give than to receive" (Acts 20:35).

But what does giving money have to do with addiction? Quite a bit, actually. When you give to others, three things happen.

1. Your focus becomes outward, rather than inward.
2. You grow in your spiritual life.
3. You develop habits of obedience to God.

The opposite is also true. By keeping your money, you are inward focused, drift in your spiritual life, and you live outside of God's perfect plan.

No matter how much you have, you can give something. Start giving. Start small. Start today.

Week 45
Amends

*"If actions were always judged by their consequence,
we'd spend half our lives making amends."*

- Luke Skywalker

THIS WEEK'S EXERCISE
Make Amends

In 12-Step work, we don't make amends until the 9th Step. And that's a problem. It is not healthy—for us or the other person—to wait too long to make amends. And that was never the intent by the authors of the 12 Steps. They actually meant for the Steps to be completed in 30 days.

If you are in a healthy place, regardless of where you are in your Step work, now is a good time to make amends. Your spouse or child shouldn't have to wait several months to hear your remorse, apology, and intent to live a better life.

By the time you have come to this exercise, you have probably already been in recovery for a while. You may have completed my 90-Day Recovery or some lesser plan (humor intended). So you have likely already made some amends.

We will not try to get into the details of making amends here. For that, I suggest reading my 90-Day Recovery Guide or other literature. For this week's purposes, let's not make this too difficult. Ask God to impress you with the name of one person to whom you can make amends, and then schedule a time to do this. Your amends should be in writing, and read to this person. Write a rough draft below.

Name of the person to whom I will make amends: _____

My relationship with this person: _____

When I will attempt to make amends: _____

I did it! These are my reflections on making amends with this person: _____

_____

_____

_____

_____

_____

Rough Draft of My Amends

_____

_____

_____

_____

_____

_____

_____

_____

_____

_____

Day 1
Amends

When working the 12 Steps, many men and women hit the wall with Steps eight and nine. These Steps tell us to "make a list of all persons we have harmed and become willing to make amends to them all," and then to "make direct amends to such people wherever possible, except when to do so would injure them or others."

Many times, making amends is about keeping promises made years before. King David did this in regard to his friend Jonathan. David had made a covenant to bless Jonathan's family (1 Samuel 20:14-17), but failed to fulfill this promise. Years later, after the deaths of both Saul and his son Jonathan, David knew he needed to make amends for his failure to live up to his commitments. So he asked around, "Is anyone in Saul's family still alive—anyone to whom I can show kindness for Jonathan's sake?" (2 Samuel 9:1). He was directed to Mephibosheth, Jonathan's son.

David not only hosted Mephibosheth for a banquet at the king's table, where he would eat the king's food; he declared, "I will give you all the property that once belonged to your grandfather Saul" (9:3).

That's some serious amends making! So what about you? In your addiction, you have a past littered with broken promises. It is never too late to make amends, either directly to the person you have hurt, or, as in the case of Mephibosheth, to someone else.

Day 2
Restitution

Restitution—it's something we don't talk about much, and we do it even less. But restitution is a key to recovery. Restitution is a biblical word for making amends. And the concept is rooted in the Law of Moses.

One of the earliest writings of the Law includes a passage on making restitution.

"They must confess the sin they have committed. They must make full restitution for the wrong they have done, add a fifth of the value to it and give it all to the person they have wronged" (Numbers 5:7).

God provided clear steps for those who have violated others. These steps include admitting the wrong things we have done and providing restitution wherever possible. If we follow these simple steps, we will make significant progress toward recovery.

There are three ways to make amends.

First, we can make direct amends—to the person we have offended, in an effort to make things right. Sometimes, it is not possible or wise to contact the offended party. In these cases, we can make indirect amends—doing things for someone else. Finally, we can make living amends—making a lifestyle change.

It's all about restitution. In recovery, we seek to make things right. In the process, God makes us right.

Day 3
Unfinished Business

The shortest book of the New Testament tells us the story of a runaway slave named Onesimus. While in prison, Paul led Onesimus to faith in Christ. But he soon discovered that the man had fled from his master, a man named Philemon. While Onesimus was a new man in Christ, and while slavery was abhorrent, Paul sent him back to his master to surrender himself to his authority—even though his actions were punishable by death.

Paul wrote a letter to Philemon, which he stuffed in Onesimus' pocket. Imagine the surprise that must have come over Philemon when the fugitive slave returned to his estate. And imagine what went through his mind when he read the letter from Paul, an old friend.

In that letter were these words: "Onesimus is no longer like a slave to you. He is more than a slave, for he is a beloved brother" (Philemon 16).

Philemon gave Onesimus a full pardon.

Here's the lesson: your past did not disappear the moment you came to Christ or found sobriety. If you hurt people in your past, you still have unfinished business. It's called making amends. It's called doing the right thing. It's called character. Oh—and another thing. It's also called recovery.

Day 4
Dr. Simon Says

Dr. George Simon is a leading expert on manipulators and the author of *In Sheep's Clothing*. He cites four marks of true change: acknowledgment of a wrong, the willingness to confess it, the willingness to abandon it, and the willingness to make restitution.

Did you catch that last one—restitution?

When Zacchaeus—who turned government tax fraud into a sport—came to faith in Christ, it changed everything. Zacchaeus quickly raced through the first three Steps. He acknowledged that he had been robbing people of their taxes. He confessed it openly. And he committed to never doing it again. But then came the difference maker.

"Zacchaeus stood up and said to the Lord, 'Look, Lord! Here and now I give half of my possessions to the poor, and if I have cheated anybody out of anything, I will pay back four times the amount'" (Luke 19:8).

We know we have become sober because we have quit acting out. And we know we are in recovery because we make restitution. It's called *making amends*. It's the 9th Step in 12-Step work. But it doesn't have to wait. Like Zacchaeus, you can start right away.

Day 5
Amends vs. Apologies

Step 9 says, "Made direct amends to such people wherever possible, except when to do so would injure them or others."

Recovery is incomplete if it does not include amends. When most people think "amends," they confuse that for "apology." They are not the same thing.

Author Tim Stoddart explains: "There are many profound differences between giving someone an apology and making amends with them. Simply put, an apology is like putting a band aid on a wound; it covers the source of the pain until it eventually disappears. When you make a sincere apology to someone whom you have hurt, it makes you both feel better, but it doesn't really correct the situation that you created. But making amends is all about reconciliation. Making amends is the best way to reconnect with the people who have been deeply hurt as a result of your actions."

Are you willing to make amends like that?

Proverbs 14:9 reads, "Fools mock at the guilt offering, but the upright enjoy acceptance."

Guilt offerings were ordained in the Book of Leviticus. Their purpose was to express remorse for actions that injured someone else. Today, we do that with words. And this might be a good time for you to start.

Ask God to lay on your heart one person to whom you should make amends.

Day 6
December 21, 1965

It happened on December 21, 1965. The International Convention on the Elimination of All Forms of Racial Discrimination met in New York City. Representatives from every continent met, and they jointly declared an end to all forms of racial discrimination.

Problem solved.

Actually, problem not solved. But everyone felt better—for a while.

The world came together and decided that there would be no more racial discrimination. And their intentions were good. But there was no plan for follow-up, no strategy for implementation. Predictably, the great intentions, warm hugs, and fuzzy feelings did not translate into measurable results.

Similarly, millions of churches, Christ followers, and porn addicts have declared a ban on porn—from society, their homes, and their computers. Still, more people—including believers—are hooked on porn than at any other point in world history.

The Bible says, "Little children, let us not love in word or talk, but in deed and in truth" (1 John 3:18). In other words, if you have to choose between good intentions and follow-through, choose follow-through.

Day 7
Spurgeon on Recovery

On the morning of February 8, 1857, Charles Haddon Spurgeon rose to deliver his weekly sermon. His text was Psalm 19:12—"Cleanse thou me from secret faults." In his address, he said the following:

"In the Lateran Council of the Church of Rome, a decree was passed that every true believer must confess his sins, all of them, once a year to the priest. What can equal the absurdity of such a decree as that? Do they suppose that any of us can confess such a mass of sins, especially the secret sins, in the span of an hour?"

Spurgeon was right. It would be impossible for any of us to confess one year's worth of secret sins in one setting. But secrets must somehow be dealt with.

Dr. Michael Slepian, professor at Columbia, wrote *The Experience of Secrecy*. He asserts, "When people mask who they are or what they've done, they have feelings of inauthenticity that are associated with a lower quality of relationships and lower satisfaction levels in their personal lives."

If inauthenticity and lower satisfaction are what you're looking for, by all means, hang onto those secrets. Addiction counselor Nicki Nance, with Beacon College, concludes, "If your secrets drive you to relapse, and you die of your addiction, it was your secrets that killed you, not the addiction."

The opposite of recovery is secrecy. He who lives *with* secrets will die *from* secrets. And that's a terrible way to go.

Share your secrets—with your priest, pastor, counselor, sponsor, or friend. Unless you like living a life of inauthenticity and lower satisfaction.

Week 46
Persistence

"Great works are performed not by strength, but by perseverance."

\- Samuel Johnson

THIS WEEK'S EXERCISE
Draw a Picture

You need to do two things to stay sober: (a) start recovery work, and (b) continue recovery work. I wish the need for recovery work just went away. I would love to tell you that this problem will go away. For a few, it actually does. But that is rare. For most of us, this principle rings true—what it took to *get* us healthy, it will take to *keep* us healthy.

The word for the week is this—persistence.

While it's true that you may be able to back off some (no need for 90 meetings in 90 days forever), it is better to do too much recovery work than not enough.

Bud Wilkinson, the old football coach at Oklahoma, once looked up at 90,000 fans who were yelling down to the field, and said, "We have thousands of fat people in the stands telling us how to do our jobs."

To stay sober, you have to stay on the field of play. You can't let up.

For this week, you can pick between two exercises. One requires drawing, but don't let that scare you. Your work will not be graded. The other exercise will be more comfortable for those who see life as a bunch of lists.

Exercise #1

Draw a picture of what life will look like in five years, if you remain consistent in your recovery work. Be as creative as you can. Do the drawing in the space below.

Exercise #2

Make a list of the things you will commit to doing consistently for the next five years.

- _____
- _____
- _____
- _____
- _____

Day 1
Finding Nemo

Revelation 2:10 says, "Do not be afraid of what you are about to suffer. I tell you, the devil will put some of you in prison to test you, and you will suffer persecution for ten days. Be faithful, even to the point of death, and I will give you life as your victor's crown."

Paul wrote, "Do not be weary in well doing" (Galatians 6:9).

Nothing is more important to recovery than to keep doing what we know to do—over and over again. It's called persistence.

In that iconic movie *Finding Nemo*, Dory explained the key to success. "Just keep swimming. Just keep swimming. Just keep swimming, swimming, swimming. What do we do? We swim, swim, swim."

In my experience, the vast majority of those who fail in recovery fail, not for lack of knowledge, but for lack of follow through. Our problem is not that we don't know what to do, but that we don't do what we know. Success in life—and recovery—is all about persistence.

You know what to do. It's time to do what you know.

Day 2
The $1 Bike Ride

"Great job!" my granddad said as he handed me a dollar.

In one ten-minute session, my granddad taught me how to do something my dad had been trying to teach me for over a year—ride a bike without the aid of training wheels. How did he do it? He offered me a dollar. And for a 24-year-old man, that was all the motivation necessary.

Actually, I was about five. But the lesson is there either way. A reward at the end of the journey enhances the chance that journey will end well.

The same is true of recovery. While the journey itself is reward enough, the thought of hearing my Master say, "Well done, thou good and faithful servant" (Matthew 25:23) motivates me. But so does the thought of going to bed tonight absent guilt and shame.

Before I made it around the block the first time, I fell a few times. The result was two skinned knees and one bruised ego. But I kept at it, because the reward of success was worth it.

The same is true in recovery. If you've fallen, get back up. Stay at it and your progress will lead to victory—and a good reward at the end of the journey, as well as at the end of today.

Day 3
Stay at It

Charles Schultz debuted his first-ever Peanuts comic strip on October 2, 1950, in nine newspapers around America. Over the next six decades, Schultz produced 18,000 more comic strips. The wisdom of Charlie Brown, Lucy, Linus, and the whole gang has guided many of us through the challenges of life.

One of those challenges—especially for those of us in recovery—is to stay at the hard work necessary to find success. We give up too early.

Lucy has the answer. "If no one answers the phone, dial louder."

Paul said it like this. "To those who by persistence in doing good seek glory, honor and immortality, he will give eternal life" (Romans 2:7).

One day a young lady was driving with her dad in the passenger seat. They encountered a bad storm. She noticed that several cars had pulled over because of the severity of the storm. She asked, "Should I pull over?" Her dad said to keep driving. The storm got worse, and more cars pulled over. "Should I pull over now?" asked the young driver. "No, keep driving," said her dad. Eventually, they emerged from the storm. "Now pull over," said the father. "Why now?" asked his daughter. "So you can look back at all the people who gave up and are still in the storm."

The fact is, the road to recovery will encounter many storms. The answer is not to pull over, but to keep driving. It's about persistence. It's about determination.

Day 4
Toe Stubs

Charles Kettering, CEO at General Motors, observed, "You never stub your toe when you are standing still."

The wisest man of the Old Testament was never one to stand still. Solomon was an advocate for taking risks and moving forward when all signs point the other way.

Solomon wrote, "He who observes the wind will not sow and he who regards the clouds will not reap" (Ecclesiastes 11:4).

The king's message was profound. If we only run when the wind is at our backs, we will die standing still.

Recovery will *always* demand a sprint into the wind. As Seneca said, "It's not because things are difficult that we dare not venture. It's because we dare not venture that they are difficult."

The task of recovery is hard, but the cost of failure is greater.

If you are to maintain sobriety, you will have to attend meetings when you don't feel like it, pray when you are exhausted, and reject invasive thoughts when you are in your weakest moments.

Day 5
Go Long

The longest movie ever filmed was *Ambiance*, at a remarkable 720 hours. The longest banana split was built by college students at Texas A&M, in 2018. It was 4,549 feet long. The longest baseball game was played on May 8, 1984, and lasted 33 innings. The world's longest river is the Amazon, at nearly 4,000 miles.

Going long is a good thing—especially in recovery. Scripture says, "Therefore, since we are surrounded by such a great cloud of witnesses, let us throw off everything that hinders and the sin that so easily entangles. And let us run with perseverance the race marked out for us, fixing our eyes on Jesus, the pioneer and perfecter of our faith" (Hebrews 12:1-2).

Napoleon called endurance the "greatest virtue" of a soldier. And Virgil said, "Come what may, all bad fortune must be conquered by endurance."

To find—and then secure—recovery, you have to go long. There are two times in your recovery journey when you will not make it without great endurance.

1. When you get started
2. When you keep going

Let me make it really simple. To win the race, you only need to do one thing. Keep running.

If you are new to recovery, embrace endurance. If you've been at this a while, embrace endurance. That's the only way you will ever cross the finish line—by going long.

Day 6
The Oldest Olympian Ever

It happened in 1932. Winslow Homer became the oldest Olympian in history—at the age of 96. This is his story.

Until 1952, Olympic medals were awarded in such non-athletic categories as literature, music, sculpture, and city planning. On July 30, 1932, Winslow Homer, the American painter known for his rich seascapes, became the world's oldest Olympian when his watercolor *Casting* was entered into the painting event of the Summer Games in Los Angeles.

Homer was also deceased at the time, making him not only the oldest Olympian competitor—at 96 years, 157 days—but the only dead one, too.

History is replete with old guys who made it big. George Foreman won the heavyweight title at 45, Alexander Fleming discovered penicillin at 47, Mark Twain wrote *Huckleberry Finn* at 49, and Morgan Freeman's first Hollywood role came at age 52. Colonel Sanders founded KFC at 65, Peter Roget invented the thesaurus at 73, and Fauja Singh ran his first marathon when he was 90.

Paul wrote, "We do not lose heart. Though outwardly we are wasting away, yet inwardly we are being renewed day by day" (2 Corinthians 4:16).

Here's the lesson: you are never too old to get well. I have a friend who did not find sobriety until age 92. So don't lose heart. Your best days are still in front of you.

Day 7
Good Grief

In one day, Job lost his servants, animals, and all of his offspring. Then he was afflicted with painful sores from head to toe. Before it was over, his loss and pain were immeasurable.

How did God respond? With silence. It was not until the 38th chapter of Job that God even showed up, when "the Lord spoke to Job out of the storm" (38:1).

What's with that? Before God restored Job to his former greatness—and more—he gave him time to grieve.

We must not understate the blessing of grief. It is in these storms of life that we seek God from desperate hearts. And then we wait.

Ralph Waldo Emerson wrote, "A hero is no braver than an ordinary man, but he is brave five minutes longer."

Perhaps you have experienced ridiculous pain—from abuse, trauma, or isolation. You may be a betrayed spouse. You feel lonely and lost, exhausted and exasperated, hopeless and helpless.

Here's the answer. When you feel like quitting, keep going. When you can't take another step, walk with God. He always shows up, he always answers, and he always heals every pain—at just the right time.

Week 47
Anger

*"For every minute you remain angry, you give
up sixty seconds of peace of mind."*

\- Ralph Waldo Emerson

THIS WEEK'S EXERCISE
Rate Yourself

A friend who has been a counselor for 35 years told me that he believes that anger is at the root of all addiction. That made me mad! Now, I'm no psychologist, and I certainly don't have the training necessary to either support or refute my friend's analysis. But we all know that anger is a huge component of addiction. This anger may be directed at ourselves, someone else, or even God. And we all have it—on some level.

When I hear anger in an addict's voice, I know what is probably coming next. Relapse follows anger like wet follows rain. They are pretty hard to separate.

So let's dig a little deeper. Think about a recent bout with anger, then journal about how it affected your sobriety, below.

Date of your anger: _____

How much anger did you feel (scale of 1-10)? _____

What happened to make you angry? _____

_____

_____

_____

_____

_____

_____

Did you act out sexually as a result? _____

How did you feel after this bout with anger? _____

_____

_____

_____

_____

What are you going to do differently the next time you feel anger coming on? ___

_____

_____

_____

Day 1
Anger Management

Anger is one of the strongest triggers of inappropriate behavior. In 12-Step meetings, we often hear of the "big four" known as H.A.L.T. We are at our greatest risk when we are *hungry, angry, lonely,* or *tired.*

Untreated anger makes true recovery impossible. Anger gives birth to bitterness, and bitterness blocks healthy progress.

Paul understood the danger of anger when he wrote to the church, "In your anger do not sin" (Ephesians 4:26).

Ridding ourselves of anger is not always easy. Mark Twain's strategy was simple: "When angry, count to four. When very angry, swear."

Colin Powell said, "Get mad, then get over it."

But anger is not something we just "get over." It is like our other character defects. Anger must be surrendered to God. You can do that today. Tell God about your anger, and ask him to remove it, just like every other defect that stands in the way of sobriety and recovery.

Day 2
All the Rage

Most addicts have anger issues. Some of us have a history of rage, so we try to stifle our feelings. Others stuff their feelings of anger, pretending they don't exist. Why? We were never allowed to express these feelings in the past. Evaluating our anger and how to deal with it appropriately is an important part of our recovery.

We are warned in Scripture to be "slow to anger" (James 1:19).

Why is this important in recovery? Because anger leads to bitterness, and bitterness leads to fall. Our anger hurts those around us, but it mostly hurts us.

Ralph Waldo Emerson wrote, "For every minute you remain angry, you give up sixty seconds of peace of mind."

That's sixty seconds you cannot afford to give up.

Early in my recovery, I was angry toward those who contributed to my childhood isolation. I was angry toward family, neighbors, friends—and God. Especially God. But through therapy and growth, I learned to deal with my anger. It's not that anger ever really goes away, but it can be managed. Let's rephrase that. *It must be managed.*

Day 3
Beyond Victimhood

Whether you are the victim of abuse, trauma, or isolation—which led you into a life of addiction, or have been victimized by your spouse's illicit behavior, you will never recover until you make that most difficult decision—move beyond victimhood.

Let me be provocative. When you are stuck in blame, you are stuck in victim. In other words, when you keep your eyes on the source of your pain, they cannot be on the source of your healing.

Dr. Kevin Carlsmith, professor of social psychology at Colgate University, spoke of what he called "the diminishing return of blame." Carlsmith explains, "Rather than providing closure, blame does the opposite. It keeps the wound open and fresh."

The clinicians at Learning Minds are even more direct. In an article titled *Six Signs You May Have a Victim Mentality*, they write, "Stop being entitled! Guess what—the world owes you nothing, not a thing, not even a sandwich. So stop crying about your entitlement and get out there and work for something. This will give you a push and it will show you what the world really is—an indifferent rock on which we spin round and round."

Are those words too harsh? Probably. But don't miss the bigger point. As long as you live the life of a victim, you will not know the life of a victor.

The Bible says, "In all these things, we are more than conquerors" (Romans 8:37). The sooner we believe that—and live like it—the sooner we will get well.

Day 4
Anger

Anger will never get you where you want to be.

It is natural for an addict to be angry. There's the dad who first exposed him to porn. There's the neighbor who crossed sexual boundaries. There's the wife who withheld sex for years. There's the impulse that wouldn't go away. Of course he's angry. But anger is always the enemy of recovery.

Anger will never get you where you want to be.

It is also natural for the spouse to be angry. She didn't ask for this. If only her husband had been honest about his issues before they got married. If only her counselor had given better advice. If only the children didn't have to go through all the turmoil.

Anger will never get you where you want to be.

All anger is justified on some level. That's why it's so easy to embrace. But the Bible warns, "In your anger do not sin. Do not let the sun go down while you are still angry. Do not give the devil a foothold" (Ephesians 4:26-27). I can't solve your anger issues with a short column. That's why God created therapists. If you battle anger, you're in trouble. So seek help today.

Day 5
Family of Origin

It was a great tipping moment for the children of God. The Jewish exiles, now returning to their homeland, "confessed their own sins and the sins of their ancestors" (Nehemiah 9:2).

Don't miss that last part—"and the sins of their ancestors." Family history matters. What our ancestors did went a long way in determining who we would become.

Let's dig a little deeper. The Israelites blamed their years of captivity on their ancestors. They said, "Our ancestors refused to turn from their wickedness. So now today we are slaves in the land of plenty that you gave them for their enjoyment. We serve conquering kings at their pleasure, and we are in great misery" (Nehemiah 9:35-37).

It is sometimes necessary to trace the roots of our slavery to addiction. As for me, my therapist has helped me trace some unseen influences back to a grandfather I never knew. Our families of origin play huge roles in who we become.

However, we cannot blame our ancestors for the choices we make today. Our relatives may be partly responsible for bringing us to this point, but we are wholly responsible for moving to a better place.

Day 6
It's What Dummies Do

The smartest man (Solomon) had strong words for the dumbest man (any of us). "Fools give full vent to their rage" (Proverbs 29:11).

That's pretty rough. Solomon calls those who cannot control their anger "fools."

Here's one of the biggest problems with anger: it leads to—and often even becomes—another addiction.

Dr. Jean Kim writes, "What happens is that anger can lead to similar 'rushes' as thrill-seeking activities where danger triggers dopamine reward receptors in the brain, like other forms of addiction."

Those who understand sex addiction will recognize that word *dopamine*.

Addiction is often recognized (and disguised) by anger. So take your anger issues seriously. As bad as anger can be, when left untreated, it leads to all kinds of other problems.

You will never enjoy lasting sobriety until you deal with your anger issues. And there is no better time to start than today.

Day 7
Make Anger Work for You

We have spent the last week criticizing anger. There is a reason for that. Anger—when left untreated—can lead to addiction, break up marriages, and destroy lives.

But what if we make anger work *for* us instead of *against* us? Let me explain. If you respond to your periods of anger, instead of trying to ignore them, three productive outcomes may result.

1. Self-improvement
2. Course correction
3. Renewed recovery

The editorial staff of American Addiction Centers writes, "Anger is not necessarily bad, as all emotions have functional attributes." In other words, God can take your anger and turn it into something positive.

Often, the genesis of anger is fear—of the past or future. Theologian Groucho Marx said, "Yesterday is dead, tomorrow hasn't arrived yet. I have just one day—today—and I'm going to be happy in it."

"Anger does not produce the righteousness that God desires" (James 1:20).

You can't avoid anger altogether. But what you can do is learn from it—then let it go. Until you learn to control your anger, your anger will control you.

Week 48
Regrets

"Make the most of your regrets."

- Henry David Thoreau

THIS WEEK'S EXERCISE
Face Your Regrets

Anyone who says they have no regrets hasn't lived very long. Or their memory is really bad. Or they have a heart of stone. We all have regrets. We have things we wish we could do over. I've never met a person who, if he could live his life over, wouldn't change a thing.

The problem with regrets isn't that we have them, but that we haven't learned from them. Our regrets can be really good teachers. The only way your past mistakes win is if you let them. Any experience we learn from can be turned into a positive. When Paul promised that "all things work together for good to those who love God" (Romans 8:28), he didn't limit these things to "good things." He said, "all things."

List three regrets of your past, and more importantly, what you can learn from them or how you can make them right.

Regret #1: _____

What I can learn from it or do to fix it: _____

_____

Regret #2: _____

What I can learn from it or do to fix it: _____

_____

Regret #3: _____

What I can learn from it or do to fix it: _____

_____

Day 1
When You Are Overwhelmed

King David prayed, "Though we are overwhelmed by our sins, you forgive them all" (Psalm 65:3).

The life of King David gives us hope. He had committed sins that would get any pastor fired, any president impeached, and any other person sued. But when he came to his senses, he came to his God. First overwhelmed by his sins, he became overwhelmed by God's grace.

Dorothy Hamill said, "At times I feel overwhelmed and my depression leads me into darkness."

John Calvin wrote, "Seeing that a Pilot steers the ship in which we sail, who will never allow us to perish even in the midst of shipwrecks, there is no reason why our minds should be overwhelmed with fear and overcome with weariness."

Perhaps you have driven your "ship" into the darkest, most stormy waters. But it is in the desperation of your darkest moment that God shines his brightest light. Do you feel overwhelmed by sin, guilt, and shame? That's okay—God is about to do what he does best.

If you are feeling overwhelmed by the mistakes of the past, confess that to the one who stands ready to overwhelm you with the forgiveness of all eternity.

Day 2
Cat's in the Cradle

When the Bible speaks of a father's sin affecting the second and third generation, this was because in those days, three generations lived together. Our children become who we are, not who we want them to be.

In his iconic song, *Cat's in the Cradle*, Harry Chapin wrote this famous last stanza:

I've long since retired and my son's moved away.
I called him up just the other day.
I said, "I'd like to see you if you don't mind."
He said, "I'd love to, dad, if I could find the time.
You see, my new job's a hassle,
And the kids have the flu.
But it's sure nice talking to you, dad.

It's been sure nice talking to you."
And as I hung up the phone, it occurred to me,
He'd grown up just like me.
My boy was just like me.

Attend any 12-Step meeting, and you will hear something like this: "I discovered my dad's pornography when I was nine years old." The fact is, our kids are watching—and learning. Keep that in mind the next time you are tempted to act out.

Our children will tend to be like us, not like we want them to be. So take one step today to become the person you want them to be.

Day 3
The Gift of Pain

If you have avoided the consequences of bad choices, I'm sorry. This is bad news. If you have had multiple affairs, become addicted to porn, or engaged in chronic masturbation, but it hasn't cost you anything, you have my deepest sympathies.

Here's the deal—until we feel pain, we rarely get well. C.S. Lewis called pain "God's great unwanted gift." And addiction specialist Dr. Craig Cashwell says, "The number one motivation for change is pain."

It has been my observation that very few go all in with recovery until their addiction has cost them dearly. Until they have lost their marriage, health, job, or reputation, they try to live in two worlds. They want to have it both ways.

We have this promise from God: "He heals the brokenhearted and binds up their wounds" (Psalm 147:3).

This is a great promise, but it's not an unconditional promise. God only heals those who come to him in their brokenness. And most of us don't go to the doctor, let alone the Great Physician, until we are really sick. Very few of us turn from destructive addictions until we feel significant pain. I pray you will be the exception.

You can wait to get help after your addiction ruins everything. Or you can get to work on recovery now. It's your call.

Day 4
Chariots of Fire

Conviction. Let's talk about it. Thomas Carlyle said, "Conviction is worthless unless it is converted into conduct." What does this look like? I suggest it looks a lot like Eric Liddell, the subject of the movie, *Chariots of Fire.*

In one pivotal scene the Scottish runner tried to explain to members of the British Olympic committee why he couldn't race on Sundays. It was because of his faithfulness to God, who commanded believers to honor the Sabbath.

Eric Liddell stayed true to his convictions, and he still won a gold medal at the 1924 Olympics. While he treasured the award, it was his next chapter in life that meant more to him. Liddell became a missionary to China, where he died at the young age of 43.

G.K. Chesterton said, "Courage is almost a contradiction in terms. It means a strong desire to live, taking the form of a readiness to die."

Here's my conclusion of the matter. God calls few of us to die for our convictions. But he calls all of us to have convictions worth dying for.

That's how Paul lived his life. He knew the price he was about to pay for following Christ, which is why he told dear friends, "I know that none of you among whom I have gone about preaching the kingdom will ever see me again" (Acts 20:25).

It's time that your desires became convictions. And it's time for your convictions to become action.

Day 5
Never Alone

In the United States, there are 400,000 children living in foster care. One-fourth of those are ready to be adopted, but there aren't enough parents to take in all these precious children.

Our sin has left us as orphans, separated from God. But fortunately, he is in the adoption business. As my pastor likes to say, "Jesus was, is, and always will be a come as you are Savior. But he never was and never will be a leave you as you are Lord."

The goal is transformation. The means is connection. When we connect with God and walk with him we find the strength to overcome.

Jesus promised his followers, "I will not leave you as orphans; I will come to you" (John 14:18).

When the great John Wesley was asked to reflect on the benefits of God, he said, "The best thing of all is God is with us."

We all have something wrong with us. And regardless of the problem, the solution is the same.

God's love is unconditional and always waiting for us. Turning our life and will over to God involves opening the door of our heart to his love. Filling up on God's love helps us to avoid relapses. It meets us at our deepest need and overcomes our most powerful insecurities.

Claim the foundational promise to recovery—you are not alone.

Day 6
David and Goliath

The story of David and Goliath is one for the ages. In fact, it is one for *all ages*. We all love the story of the little, good guy who beat the big, bad guy. But there's something missing from the story that I bet you never noticed.

God never actually told David to fight Goliath.

There is something in our youth that is willing to risk, to go all in. We feel we can climb the highest mountain and defeat the strongest foe. Then we grow up.

You can err in one of two ways—doing too little or doing too much. I like the way Lucille Ball said it: "I'd rather regret the things I've done than the things I haven't done."

Overcoming unhealthy behaviors does not mean adopting a passive mindset. To the contrary, sobriety will be your greatest challenge, recovery your most noble adventure.

Attaining a sober, balanced, healthy life is not for the weak of heart. Recovery is reserved only for those who are willing to go all in. It's not easy, but it is necessary.

Day 7
In Light of Death

Nothing puts life in perspective like death.

Steve Jobs said, "Remembering that I'll be dead soon is the most important tool I've ever encountered to help me make the big choices in life."

The Bible says, "A good person dies, and so does a sinner" (Ecclesiastes 9:2).

Like most of us, I didn't think much about death as a young man. But the humbling truth is that many actually die—as young men. Consider the age at which these people died: Anne Frank (15), Richie Valens (17), Buddy Holly (22), James Dean (24), Janis Joplin (27), Jimi Hendrix (27), Hank Williams (29), Jim Croce (30), Karen Carpenter (32), Darryl Kile (33), John Belushi (33), Princess Diana (36), Marilyn Monroe (36), Lou Gehrig (37), John F. Kennedy, Jr. (38), Martin Luther King, Jr. (39).

When I think of the uncertainty of life and the certainty of death, it affects the way I view life, especially in light of my addiction. I know that I am closer to my death than ever before. Knowing that I will die, and that it could be soon (sounds morbid, but it's true) changes everything: my plans, priorities, and perspective.

What about you? If you knew you were going to die tomorrow, would you make different choices today? I'm guessing you would.

Week 49
Realignment

"To improve is to change; to be perfect is to change often."

\- Winston Churchill

THIS WEEK'S EXERCISE
Listen to This

From time to time, it is wise to reevaluate our recovery. Are we on the right track? Have we fallen into a rut? Are we still growing in our spiritual walk? Are we still moving forward in our sobriety? Have we learned anything new than can help us maintain recovery for life?

It is good to listen to a new voice occasionally. One way to do that is by listening to a podcast on recovery. There are many options available. I will list a few ministries that provide excellent podcasts. Feel free to find your own podcast. After you listen to this podcast, write your reflections below. Look for one significant lesson or principle that applies to your own recovery.

Podcasts that will bless your recovery:

- Pure Sex Radio (2.bebroken.com)
- Castimonia (castimonia.org)
- Porn-Free Radio (recoveredman.com)
- Carol the Coach (sexhelpwithcarolthecoach.com)
- XXXChurch (xxxchurch.com)
- Bethesda Workshops (bethesdaworkshops.org)
- Prodigal's International (prodigalsinternational.org)

Date I listened to a podcast: _____

The podcast I listened to: _____

Lessons/principles I heard that will help my personal recovery:

- _____
- _____
- _____

Day 1
Realignment

Charlie Brown commented on what it meant to have a good day. "I know it's going to be a good day when all the wheels on my shopping cart turn the same way."

If ever there was a time when our lives needed to be in alignment, it is in our personal recovery. That means having all our wheels headed in the same direction—therapy, meetings, prayer, working the Steps, calling our sponsor, surrender, honesty. If we try to maintain sobriety with even one of the wheels out of alignment, we will live a life of constant frustration.

The good news is the road to recovery is well-lit. "The Lord says, 'I will guide you along the best pathway for your life'" (Psalm 32:8). God is committed to your personal recovery.

Martin Luther King, Jr., said, "Faith is taking the first step, even when you don't see the whole staircase."

When I got into recovery, I didn't see the whole staircase. But I always saw the next step. And that is enough.

Be proactive. Do the things that keep your cart headed in the right direction. Follow God's plan for your life—one day at a time.

Day 2
Time to Fly

Larry Walker wanted to fly. It was his greatest passion and dream. Not born with wings, he had to become rather creative. So he hitched up 45 helium-filled balloons to his lawn chair. He strapped himself in, with a snack, soft drink, and pellet gun. His plan was to rise 30 feet into the air, then shoot the balloons to bring about a slow, gentle landing.

He overshot his target. Larry's lawn chair rocketed to heights of 16,000 feet! He then shot his balloons until he landed in some power lines. When arrested, he told the police, "A man can't just sit there."

Recovery is nothing more than redirected passion. It calls us to a universe where the impossible becomes possible, the unimaginable reality.

We really can be free! We can fly—above circumstances, temptations, and our past. But it starts with a passion to go where we have not been and to do what we have not tried.

Yogi Berra said it like this: "If all you do is what you've done, all you'll get is what you've got."

God said it like this, speaking to Moses: "The Lord had said to Moses, 'Leave your country, your people and your father's household and go to the land I will show you'" (Genesis 12:1).

God has big plans. You've been grounded by your addiction long enough. It's time to fly.

Day 3
Change

About 2500 years ago, Chinese philosopher Lao Tzu said, "If you do not change direction, you may end up where you are headed."

Progress requires change.

The prince of prophets said, "See, I am doing a new thing! Now it springs up; do you not perceive it? I am making a way" (Isaiah 43:19).

The easy way out is to change your circumstances. But that rarely works. That leaves us with the real solution to recovery. In the words of Victor Frankl, "When we are no longer able to change a situation, we must change ourselves."

I suggest you pray the Serenity Prayer every day. Don't miss the second part of the prayer: "God grant me the serenity to accept the things I cannot change, *the courage to change the things I can,* and the wisdom to know the difference."

Gandhi said, "You must be the change you wish to see." That can start today. Submit to the one who promised, "I am doing a new thing!"

Day 4
Double Life

Chad worked hard and usually came straight home after work. But once a month, he stopped by a massage parlor on the way home. Sue taught a children's dance class. There, she met Jeff, the father of one of her students, and a six-month affair ensued. Sam traveled to Chicago once every few weeks on business. There, he met a prostitute, whom he paid for sex for three years.

Bill W., one of the founders of AA, said, "More than most people, the addict lives a double life. He is very much the actor."

I've never met an addict who didn't live a double life. In fact, I'm not sure I've ever met *anyone* who didn't live a double life on some level. Who we are on stage rarely matches who we are back stage.

And that gets us into trouble. James said, "A person with divided loyalty is as unsettled as a wave of the sea that is blown and tossed by the wind" (James 1:7).

The essence of recovery is bringing these two lives into alignment. And one of the best places to do that is in a recovery group. Okay, I'm thinking it, so I'll say it. I find more honesty in an SA group than I do in most Sunday school groups. It is there that the double life is exposed, not hidden. And the healing begins.

Are you living a double life? Does the person you present on stage match who you are back stage? If not, it's time to get real, be honest, and surround yourself with others committed to the same ideals.

Day 5
Buy Ducks

There was a chicken farmer whose land was flooded every spring. He didn't want to give up his farm, but when the water backed up onto his land and flooded his chicken coops, it was always a struggle to get his chickens to higher ground. Some years he couldn't move fast enough and hundreds of his chickens drowned.

After his worst spring ever, and having lost his entire flock, he came into his farmhouse and said to his wife, "I've had it. I can't afford to buy another place. I can't sell this one. I don't know what to do."

His wife offered the obvious: "Buy ducks."

Author Neale Donald Walsh asserted, "Life begins at the end of your comfort zone."

Perhaps you've been through a few floods in your life. The good news for the farmer is that he had his wife. And she told him to make something great from what seemed to be a disaster. God does the same for you. From the floods can come great victory. But only if you don't try to go it alone.

Moses encountered his share of difficulties. He offered this promise: "He [God] is the one who goes before you. He will be with you. He will not leave you or forsake you. Do not be afraid" (Deuteronomy 31:8).

When tough times come, keep moving forward. But don't do it alone.

Day 6
Change You Can Believe In

Lucy announced to Charlie Brown, "I'm going to change the world. I think I'll start with you."

In recovery, we seek to change our spouse, our kids, our boss, and our circumstances. But the only person we can really change is the one looking at us in the mirror every time we brush our teeth.

Rumi, a 13th-century Persian theologian, said, "Yesterday I was clever, so I wanted to change the world. Today, I am wise, so I am changing myself."

Recovery is all about change. But it is only about changing yourself.

Jeff Bridges, who has battled alcohol abuse, said, "The way to change the world is by taking responsibility for yourself."

To defeat your problem you must first own your problem. Then you must own your change. People can change, but they can only change themselves. So quit worrying about everyone else and focus on yourself. As Jesus said in the Denison Translation of the Bible, "Get the telephone pole out of your own eye before you worry about the speck in your neighbor's eye" (Matthew 7:5).

Recovery requires change. That change begins and ends with you. Take the steps of change that bring recovery, and leave everyone else to God.

Day 7
Lesson from Yoda

Yoda, the Star Wars Jedi Master, was a great life coach. In *The Empire Strikes Back*, he challenged Luke Skywalker to shift his mindset from self-limiting thoughts to one of possibilities, with these famous words:

"You must unlearn what you have learned."

Lao Tzu, the Chinese philosopher from 2,500 years ago, said it like this: "To attain knowledge, add things every day. To attain wisdom, subtract things every day."

To find success in life is not just a matter of addition. It also includes subtraction.

For example, in recovery, you need to unlearn the following precepts that guided your life for too long: "I can do this in my own strength." "I can stop anytime." "I don't need anyone else's help." "This thing I keep doing over and over, year after year after year—it's not really an addiction."

Jesus warned against using a new cloth to sew an old garment or pouring new wine into old wineskins (Matthew 9:14-17). In recovery, we cannot find success by using the same old "cloths" and "wineskins" that got us into trouble in the first place.

Recovery is about embracing new ideas and principles that work. But first, we must unlearn what we've already learned.

Be willing to let go of some old ideas. Why? Because they didn't work.

Week 50
Patience

"He that can have patience can have what he will."

- Benjamin Franklin

THIS WEEK'S EXERCISE
Get Two Chairs

We often become impatient with our recovery. Everyone wants to be *recovered*, but no one wants to be *recovering*. With time, it gets easier. The euphoric recall, fantasies, and triggering thoughts slowly diminish. We develop new habits and become stronger. With each small step forward, we find ourselves progressively overcoming our worst demons.

Recovery cannot be rushed. It is a marathon, with a lot of hurdles along the way. But recovery will come if we stay at it.

You can be light years ahead of where you are now, in one year. But that will only happen if you make wise choices now. You can't just wake up one day and live in freedom any more than you can wake up one day—50 pounds overweight—and decide to run a marathon that afternoon.

To be well in one year, you must focus on the things you can do today. This exercise will require four things:

- Two chairs
- A quiet room
- This workbook
- A pen

Get that set up, and you can go to work.

Step 1—Sit in one of the chairs, facing the other chair, with this workbook in hand.

Step 2—Write down five things you will change in the coming year. These may include doing 12-Step work, joining a group, reading a book, getting on Covenant Eyes, getting a sponsor, seeing a therapist, or going through my 90-Day Recovery Plan. Get creative. Write this down below.

1. _____

2. _____

3. _____

4. _____

5. _____

Step 3—Imagine your life in one year, if you complete all of these five tasks. Now go sit in the opposite chair—which represents your life in one year—and thank God in advance for what is to come.

Day 1
Green Apples

Playwright Alice Chapin wrote, "How could I possibly be the apple of God's eye when my behavior is not yet perfect? Because green apples are apples, too. One day I shall be a mature September apple, perfectly formed. But for now, I am still growing."

God's love transcends man's shortcomings. He promises, "I have loved you with an everlasting love; therefore, I have continued my faithfulness to you" (Jeremiah 31:3).

One of the keys to recovery is patience. God is at work in us, whether we see it or not. And he works on his terms and in his timing.

Phillips Brooks, the famous New England pastor of the late 1800s, was once spotted pacing the floor like a caged animal. A friend asked him what was wrong. Brooks responded, "The trouble is I'm in a hurry, but God is not!"

Step Four talks about character defects. We all have them, but God is still at work. And if we are faithful to our work, God will be faithful to his. Change will come—if we are patient.

Day 2
Learn from the Snail

Nineteenth century preacher Charles Spurgeon taught what he called "the lesson of the snail." He said, "By perseverance the snail reached the ark."

Nothing will bring you victory over lust like perseverance. Never give up. Failure is the path of least persistence.

Consider the honey bee. To produce one pound of honey he must visit 56,000 clover heads. Since each head has 60 flower tubes, he must make 3.36 million visits to produce one pound of honey.

A Little League baseball team trailed by 21 runs entering the bottom of the first inning. Still, one of the players remained confident. "Why are you so optimistic?" a coach asked. "It's simple," said the boy. "We haven't batted yet."

Lust. A second look. Fantasy. We all battle these temptations—and more. And none of us has been victorious every time. But that's okay. The key to victory is perseverance. Stay in the battle. Keep swinging.

Your job is simple. Do the next right thing. Then do that again tomorrow. Take small steps—one day at a time. Paul said it like this: "Never tire from doing the right thing" (2 Thessalonians 3:13).

Think of yourself as the snail and the ark as recovery. You can get there. It won't be easy and it won't come fast. But it can happen—if you have perseverance.

Day 3
Humble Pie

Tax collectors were among the most despised citizens in Jewish society, whereas Pharisees were the most respected. Jesus was cognizant of this reality when he made a hero out of a tax collector in the following story.

"Two men went to the Temple to pray. One was a Pharisee, and the other was a despised tax collector. The Pharisee stood by himself and prayed this prayer: 'I thank you, God, that I am not like other people—cheaters, sinners, adulterers. I'm certainly not like that tax collector!' But the tax collector beat his chest in sorrow, saying, 'O God, be merciful to me, for I am a sinner.' I tell you, this sinner, not the Pharisee, returned home justified before God. For those who exalt themselves will be humbled, and those who humble themselves will be exalted" (Luke 18:10-14).

It is the humble heart that opens the door to God's blessing. It is when we think we have arrived that we are behind. Let me say it like this. Your past victories are no guarantee of future success.

Ernest Hemingway wrote, "There is nothing noble in being superior to your fellow man; true nobility is being superior to your former self."

Don't compare yourself to the tax collector. And don't compare yourself to the guy with less sobriety—or more. Just commit, one day at a time, to be superior to your former self.

Day 4
Saturday

"When the Sabbath was over, Mary Magdalene, Mary the mother of James, and Salome bought spices so that they might go to anoint Jesus' body" (Mark 16:1).

Tony Campolo made famous a sermon, which he first preached in Philadelphia, then around the world: "It's Friday, but Sunday's comin." Campolo contrasts how different the world looked on Friday—the day that Jesus died, as opposed to Sunday—the day of the great resurrection.

Campolo skipped one very important day in the story. We call it "Saturday." Though the other two days have earned a special place on the church calendar—Good Friday and Easter Sunday—it is Saturday where most of life is lived. Saturday represents the period after the death but before the resurrection.

Your darkest days are probably behind you, and your best days are still ahead. We can't live in the past or in the future. Life is lived today.

Andrew Murray prayed, "Father, teach us all how to wait."

Keep making good decisions day by day. Plant recovery seeds today and tomorrow will be fine. Friday has passed. Sunday will come in due time. Saturday is your gift for today. Accept it and live it.

Day 5
The Critical Component

Patience. It is a critical component of recovery. You won't get from where you are to where you want to be without it. But the recovery movement hasn't always been so accommodating.

In the 1940s, when Bill Wilson and Dr. Bob first published AA's Big Book, they encouraged their fellow alcoholics to speed through all 12 steps in their first 30 days of sobriety.

The psalmist understood the need for patience. He wrote, "I waited patiently for the Lord's help; then he listened to me and heard my cry" (Psalm 40:1).

In recovery, you will want to see the benefits of hard work immediately. But it is right practice—repeated over and over—that yields lasting change and real progress. Create a plan for the next 30 days. Include meetings, prayer, meditations, worship, exercise, and connection with others in recovery. And don't judge your progress until after the 30 days.

John Quincy Adams offered sage advice for every addict when he said, "Patience and perseverance have a magical effect before which difficulties disappear and obstacles vanish."

Do the right things today. And again tomorrow. And then, the day after that. Be patient. Recovery comes to those who wait.

Day 6
The Patient Patient

Be patient and recovery will come.

Solomon promised, "It is good to wait quietly for the salvation of the Lord" (Lamentations 3:26).

Martin Lloyd Jones said, "There is nothing which so certifies the genuineness of a man's faith as his patient endurance, his keeping on steadily in spite of everything."

We all want to recover as quickly as possible. It's hard to be patient as we wait for the process to work. Sure, we realize that we didn't get to the difficult spot we are in overnight. We understand that we cannot undo a lifetime of damage in just a few moments. But still, it is a challenge to wait patiently. But every part of the recovery process requires time and patience.

The key to tomorrow's sobriety is today's work. Attend a meeting. Call someone in the program. Read a chapter of recovery material. Pray the 3rd Step Prayer. Do the little things you can do today, and God will bring a great miracle tomorrow.

Pray the 3rd Step Prayer—"*God, I offer myself to you, to build with me and do with me as you will. Take away my difficulties, that victory over them would bear witness to those I would help of your power, your love, and your way of life.*"

Day 7
It Takes Time

The best time for you to start recovery is five years ago. The second best time is today.

Recovery requires two things—time and endurance. It comes neither quickly nor easily. But then, nothing of great value does.

Paul wrote to young Timothy: "Hardworking farmers should be the first to enjoy the fruit of their labor" (2 Timothy 2:6).

The lesson of the farmer is one of endurance. Trees are most often planted in the early spring, right after the last frost. Over the summer, water, nutrients, and sunlight will aid early growth. Results are hard to see at first, but they will come. A fast-growing tree may reach a height of 25 feet—in ten years. Apple trees take up to five years to produce apples, while cherry trees may take seven years to produce cherries.

In recovery, the results you want tomorrow will be based on the seeds you plant today. Others may not notice the changes that are taking root, but they are there. Eventually, what God is doing *in* you will be evident to those *around* you.

It's too late to write a new beginning, but it's never too late to write a new ending. You can't start your recovery five years ago, but you can start it today.

It's time to start planting.

Week 51
Memories

"One of the keys to happiness is a bad memory."

- Rita Mae Brown

THIS WEEK'S EXERCISE
Get a $10 Bill

Shame. It fills the heart of every addict. And until shame is eradicated, the addiction will generally persist, because shame says, "You are a bad person." The addict's natural response to shame is, "Well, if I'm who you say I am, I might as well continue in my destructive behaviors."

Shame is tied memories of all the bad things we have done or thought. These memories will kill us if we let them. It is critical that we understand that no matter the damage we have done to ourselves and others, we are still the redeemable creation of God. While our past may limit many opportunities for future service to the kingdom, other options will begin to open up.

Here's the deal—there is nothing you have ever done that will make God love you less.

And there's more good news—you aren't big enough to thwart God's ability to use you. At no time does God say, "Bummer! Now my son has crossed that line, and I don't know how I can ever use him again."

Here's your exercise for this week. Get ahold of a $10 bill. Any bill will work, actually, but we'll go for a $10 bill because God says you're still a "10," no matter what you've done in your past.

There are two parts to this exercise.

First, take that bill and wad it up. Bend it, fold it, roll it. Create as many creases in that $10 bill as you can.

Second, unfold the bill. Straighten it out. Now, answer the following questions.

1. Is it possible to remove all the creases and make the $10 bill look brand new again? Why or why not? _____

2. How much was the bill worth before you wadded it up? _____

_____

3. How much is it worth now? _____

391

4. What is the lesson of the $10 bill? How does this apply to your life? _____

_____

_____

Day 1
The Wedding Ring

Ravi Zacharias tells the story of a woman whose husband died. Shortly after his funeral, she lost her wedding ring. She searched everywhere, but never found it. Fifteen years later, she was working in her garden. While digging in the soil, she struck a small object buried several inches into the dirt. When she dug her hands deeper into the soil, she grabbed this piece of metal and pulled it out. To her amazement, she was holding her wedding ring in her fingers. It had been lost for a decade and a half.

Suddenly, a flood of memories overcame the widow. The ring represented a tie to her happier days. She was overcome with joy as she remembered what life had been before.

Do you remember what life was like before? Do you remember a time when you had not yet plunged into the full depths of your addiction, before you had destroyed several lives—including your own?

Let those memories serve to remind you of what life can still be like—apart from porn and sex addiction.

Isaiah spoke of a time when "the former things will not be remembered or come to mind" (Isaiah 65:17).

It's time to bury your past while unearthing your future.

Day 2
Grieving the Loss

I have a sign hanging on my wall that reads, "Your mountain is waiting, so get on your way." That is the message every addict and spouse need to hear. Yesterday's crisis opens the door to tomorrow's blessing. But we have to walk through that door.

At the age of 137, Abraham lost his beloved wife, "and Abraham went to mourn and to weep over her" (Genesis 23:2). Death brought grief. But it didn't end there. The response of Abraham is a parable for the addict and his spouse. Your addiction has killed your self-esteem, integrity, and perhaps marriage. But the story doesn't have to end there. The process of recovery can now begin.

First, there is death. When Sarah died, part of Abraham died with her. When you were discovered, it was like death. For many of us, our addiction was our closest companion.

Second, there is mourning. Abraham wept and mourned. The addict must mourn his addiction. The transition toward sobriety is one of turmoil and uncertainty . . . and a lot of pain.

Third, there must be a burial. Burying his wife was so important to Abraham that he paid 400 pieces of silver for a burial plot. The burial represents the addict's sobriety date. To get well, he must mark the final time and place he acted out.

Fourth, we must move on. Abraham lived another 38 years after Sarah's death. He even remarried. For the addict to get well, he must move on from his past. Indeed, your mountain is waiting, so get on your way.

Day 3
Short Memories

One of our biggest problems is that we have short memories. We are like the guy whose wife made him dinner every night for their entire 50 years of marriage. The next day, he asked her, "Who's cooking dinner tonight?"

God has been cooking your dinner for a long time. He has proven his faithfulness over and over. But too often, you have pulled a Rehoboam. The Bible says of the young king, "After Rehoboam's position as king was established and he had become strong, he and all Israel with him abandoned the law of the Lord" (2 Chronicles 12:1).

G.K. Chesterton recorded the following dialogue.

Father Brown: "There is one great spiritual disease."

Flambeau: "And what is the one great spiritual disease?"

Father Brown: "Thinking one is quite well."

I love the words of the old 18th century hymn, written by Isaac Watts. "When I survey the wondrous cross, on which the Prince of glory died, my richest gain I count but loss, and pour contempt on all my pride."

One of the keys to lasting recovery is to take nothing for granted. Watch out for pride. Never forget the danger of thinking you are quite well.

Day 4
Two Mice

There is a great illustration from the movie, *Catch Me If You Can*. Frank Abagnale, Sr., says, "Two little mice fell in a bucket of cream. The first mouse quickly gave up and drowned. The second mouse wouldn't quit. He struggled so hard that eventually he churned that cream into butter and crawled out. Gentlemen, as of this moment, I am that second mouse."

Every recovering addict—no matter the addiction—is that second mouse.

Daphne Rose Kingma said, "Holding on is believing that there's only a past; letting go is knowing that there's a future."

For each of us there is a past. And there is a future. But we must live in the future. Like the mouse, getting there is often a struggle. But it's worth it.

The Bible says, "Remember not the former things, nor consider the things of old. Behold, I am doing a new thing; now it springs forth, do you not perceive it? I will make a way in the wilderness and rivers in the desert" (Isaiah 43:18-19).

Think of your addiction as a bucket of cream. You can give in or you can keep fighting. It's a fight worth having. And it's a fight you can win.

Day 5
Surrendering Your Past

One of the titanic struggles in finding lasting sobriety is moving beyond our past. We know that the God who forgives our sin also forgets our sin. The problem is, we have memories that are hard to tune out. And most of us have people in our lives who are more than happy to remind us of every slip, sin, struggle, and stumble. We are haunted by our past. We remember the broken promises, false starts, and painful relapses.

As hard as it is, every person who wishes to move beyond his or her addiction, or the pain caused by another person's addiction, must learn to leave his or her past right there—in the past.

I once heard some solid advice: "When your past calls, let it go to voice mail. It has nothing to say."

Ralph Waldo Emerson framed it like this: "What lies behind us and what lies ahead of us are tiny matters compared to what lies within us."

The Apostle Paul had a checkered past, to say the least. He discovered the formula for success, in "forgetting what is behind and straining toward what is ahead" (Philippians 3:13).

You have a past. We all do. So let me say it like this. The key to a better future is to quit trying to have a better past.

You can find incredible victory. But you must learn to live in the moment. I'm not saying you can forget the past. But you can surrender it, one day at a time.

Day 6
The Proposal

The most unlikely couple in the Bible was Gomer and Hosea. Gomer (the woman) had a checkered past. But God told Hosea (the man) to pursue her anyway. And when Gomer persisted in her lifestyle as a prostitute, God gave Hosea amazing counsel.

"Go show your love to your wife again, though she is an adulteress" (Hosea 3:1). Then Hosea said to his wife, "You are to live with me many days; you must not be a prostitute or be intimate with any man, and I will behave the same way toward you" (Hosea 3:3).

God proposed that Hosea propose to his wife—a new beginning, launched from the pad of forgiveness.

We see two things here. First, adultery does not need to end a marriage. Second, sometimes, there must be a period of celibacy within the marriage so recovery can begin.

Perhaps you are a wounded spouse. You did not sign up for your mate's infidelity. And who can blame you if you file for divorce? I certainly wouldn't.

It takes a lot to stay with someone who turns out to be something less than advertised. But it's possible, and sometimes a blessing.

Marilyn Monroe said, "If you can't take me at my worst, you don't deserve me at my best."

Is the restoration of your marriage possible? Yes. Will it be easy? No. But as we say in our ministry every day, even in the face of adultery—*There's still hope.*

Day 7
Never Forget

Jim Valvano's story has inspired a generation. I still remember that awful night in Albuquerque, New Mexico. The date was April 4, 1983. North Carolina State, coached by Valvano, beat my beloved Houston Cougars for the NCAA men's basketball championship. Valvano proceeded to run all over the court looking for someone to hug. It was one of the great upsets in sports history.

Ten years later, almost to the date, Valvano lost a courageous battle with cancer at the age of 47. But it was his battle with cancer, not his success on the court, that touched millions.

Treasuring every day and knowing his fate, Coach Valvano said, "I will thank God for the day and moment I have."

What Jim Valvano did, we all must do. Never forget your blessings, and never take today's moments for granted.

Titus 3:4-5 reads, "When the kindness and love of God the Savior appeared, he saved us, not because of righteous things we had done, but because of his mercy. He saved us through the washing of rebirth and renewal by the Holy Spirit."

We all have been blessed beyond what we deserve. F.F. Bruce wrote, "God bestows his blessings without discrimination." One of the best ways to secure tomorrow's recovery is to simply thank God for the gift of today.

Week 52
Dominoes

"The domino effect has the capacity to change the course of an entire world."

- J.D. Stroube

THIS WEEK'S EXERCISE
Let's Play Dominoes

I'm going to guess that you didn't wake up one day and decide to become a sex addict. For most of us, it took years to get as messed up as we became. Addiction is the predictable result of trauma, isolation, abuse, bad choices, psychological issues, and much more. None of us will ever really know all of the components that contributed to making us who and what we are.

But most of the ingredients to our addiction are pretty clear. And they didn't all happen at once. Addiction is the culmination of events and circumstances that have taken their toll over decades of our development.

Dominoes can be used to play a game that features numbers. Or they can be set up on a table in a way that allows all of them to fall—if just one of them falls.

To find lasting freedom, you need to deal with some of the individual dominoes that have fallen in your past. Identify them below.

Childhood dominoes:

- _____
- _____
- _____

Trauma dominoes:

- _____
- _____
- _____

Abuse dominoes:

- _____
- _____
- _____

Isolation dominoes:

- _____
- _____
- _____

Relational dominoes:

- _____
- _____
- _____

Other dominoes:

- _____
- _____
- _____

Day 1
8 Minutes, 20 Seconds

It takes eight minutes and 20 seconds. That's the time required for light to travel from the sun to the earth. That means that if, for example, a huge flying saucer crashed into the sun and blew it into a million pieces (not likely), we wouldn't know about it for over eight minutes.

What does that have to do with sex addiction? That's a fair question. Let me try to connect the dots.

When someone "acts out" (porn, masturbation, affairs, prostitution, etc.), we generally address the event. What we need to focus on is the genesis of the destructive behavior. Behind every action is isolation, trauma, fantasy, and other factors we do not see. But they are the seeds that grow into the behaviors that become visible. We see everything blow up—after the real problems took root.

Novelist Richelle Goodrich writes, "Temptations don't appear nearly as harmful as the roads they lead you down."

We dabble with addictive behaviors before we indulge. It is when we fully indulge that our problem becomes known. But it was in the dabbling stage that we really needed to seek help.

The prophet said, "The soul who sins shall die" (Ezekiel 18:20). That death doesn't come quickly, but it does come.

Deal with the issues that others cannot yet see, before everything blows up.

Day 2
Dominoes

When we visited my grandparents' home in Kansas when I was a child, we spent hours playing dominoes. But I quickly found a better use for these numbered rectangles. I would collect as many of them as possible, then set them up on a large table, so that when I knocked one over, the rest would eventually fall.

It was fun to tap the first domino over, then run to the other end of the line and wait for the last one to fall. For several seconds, the last domino stood firm. But I always knew what would ultimately happen. It was going down.

That's how addiction works. Many a man or woman has relapsed by paying a prostitute, viewing pornography, masturbating, or committing some other inappropriate sexual act. When that act is over, we can't believe what just happened, and we respond in shame.

But we miss the point. The act itself is simply the last domino to fall. It is the inevitable result of a process we put in place with the first domino—a quick fantasy, a moment of lust, a flirtatious gesture. If we are to avoid future relapses, we must learn to focus on the first domino more than the last.

When Eve was confronted by God over her first sin, she said, "The serpent deceived me, and I ate" (Genesis 3:13). Eve missed the point. She left out the first domino. She only ate the forbidden fruit because she chose to listen to the serpent in the first place. She could only be deceived because she chose to listen.

Day 3
Does Porn Use Make for Better Sex?

There is a common belief that says the use of porn enhances sexual satisfaction. I'm here to explode that myth.

An extensive study was conducted of 1,500 young adults in 2018 (*Personal Pornographic Viewing and Sexual Satisfaction*, by Wright, Bridges, Sun, Ezzell, and Johnson). The study concluded that more frequent porn viewing is associated with lower sexual satisfaction. But even occasional porn viewing, just once or twice a year, results in reduction in one's sexual satisfaction within the normal context of marriage.

God's warnings about sex outside of marriage are without dispute. "The marriage bed is undefiled" (Hebrews 13:4).

God does not cross porn use off the list of acceptable behaviors because he wants us to be frustrated, but because he wants us to be happy. He made us for sex—within certain parameters. When we wander outside those parameters, we are only hurting ourselves.

So quit making excuses for your porn use. Better yet, quit using porn—not because it hurts God, but because it hurts you.

St. Augustine said, "Love God, then do whatever you please." If you are truly undecided on the whole porn issue, follow Augustine's advice. Love God, then do what suddenly seems right.

Day 4
Progressive

Jeanne Labrosse was there when Andre-Jacques Garnerin became the first person to jump from a hydrogen balloon in a parachute, in 1797. Two years later, on October 12, 1799, Labrosse became the first woman to parachute from a balloon, jumping from a height of 3,000 feet.

First, Labrosse was content to watch someone else jump from a balloon. Eventually, after watching others jump on ten different occasions, the urge overcame her, and she jumped herself.

That's called human nature. In my world, it's called addiction. As part of its definition of addiction, the American Society of Addiction Medicine states, "Without treatment or engagement in recovery activities, addiction is progressive and can result in disability or premature death."

Tim Stoddart writes, "There is no way around it. There is no way to cheat. Addiction is progressive, and it always will be."

Jesus said it like this: "Everyone who commits sin is a slave to sin" (John 8:34).

But there is hope. Recovery is hard and rigorous work. But freedom can be yours.

Day 5
A Risk Worth Taking

Every addict remembers his first 12-Step meeting. Walking into that room is one of the most courageous things he will ever do. But the essence of recovery can be summarized in the words of Erica Jong, who wrote, in *Fear of Flying*, "The trouble is, if you don't risk anything, you risk even more."

When you enter recovery, you know you may fail. But to not enter recovery is to fail already. Recovery is a risk worth taking.

Recovery is not a scientific endeavor. We stumble, trip, and sometimes fall. But we keep going. We follow the advice of Ray Bradbury: "Go to the edge of the cliff and jump off. Build your wings on the way down."

The key to victory is to keep going, no matter what.

Jesus warned, "No one who puts his hand to the plow and looks back is fit for the kingdom of God" (Luke 9:62).

Does recovery involve risk? Absolutely. But to not enter recovery is to guarantee a lifetime of destructive behaviors. Don't put recovery off until you have all the answers; that day will never come. Get started—today.

Day 6
God Wants to Drill a Man

A.W. Tozer wrote, "God never uses anyone greatly until he tests them deeply." The classic poem, *When God Wants to Drill a Man*, says it like this:

When God wants to drill a man, and thrill a man, and skill a man—to play the noblest part

When He yearns with all His heart to create so great and bold a man
That all the world shall be amazed, watch His methods, watch His ways!

How He ruthlessly perfects whom He elects! How He hammers him and hurts him, and with mighty blows converts him

Into trial shapes of clay which only God understands; while his tortured heart is crying and he lifts beseeching hands!

How He bends but never breaks when His good He undertakes; how He uses whom He chooses, and which every purpose fuses him; by every act induces him to try His splendor out. God knows what He's about.

God wants to test you, bend you, and mold you into the most amazing creation. So rejoice in what the Bible calls "the testing of your faith" (James 1:2).

Day 7
When to Start

To get well, you must get started. The enemy of recovery is not a lack of knowledge, but a lack of action. You can have all the tools in the world, but if you leave them in your toolkit, they will do you no good.

Perhaps you are waiting for the perfect feeling, time, place, and group—before you start recovery.

Russian novelist Ivan Turgenev was right: "If we wait for the moment when everything, absolutely everything is ready, we shall never begin."

Solomon said it like this: "He who observes the wind will never sow, and he who regards the clouds will not reap" (Ecclesiastes 11:4).

Caitlin McCormick writes on the regrets of older people. He cites a study by Cornell University that found that their top regret was not taking enough risks.

If you are watching recovery from the sideline, it's time to get in the game. Yes, it's hard. Yes, it involves risk. But not getting into recovery is a greater risk.

Your problem isn't that you don't know enough, but that you don't do enough. Today, that can change. Recovery is waiting for you. It's time to get going.

TEN RULES OF RECOVERY

Congratulations! You have just completed a rigorous period of recovery that will set you up for a lifetime of success. But remember, the work doesn't stop here. It's what you do next that will determine your future. You can walk in freedom from sexually compulsive activities for the rest of your life – one day at a time.

I encourage you to do two things, going forward. First, stay in a group. If you have been in one of my Freedom Groups, I hope you will keep coming back! If you are a part of some other group, keep going. You never graduate from recovery. In every meeting, you have something to learn. So stay in the fight. You are worth it!

Second, give back. If you'd like to lead others through my 90-Day Recovery Program, let me know. Perhaps God wants you to share your story, sponsor others, or write a book. One thing is for sure – what God allows, he redeems. Your story should not be kept silent. You can help others, and in the process, secure your own recovery.

One of the blessings of leading a ministry like ours is the training I have received and the hundreds of men and women we have met. I'm still learning – every day. But I want to leave you with a few things I've already learned. I call them my "Ten Rules for Recovery." I hope you'll take time to reflect on each one.

May God bless you as we continue this journey together . . .

Rule #1

God Loves me more than he hates my mess.

Rule #2

No matter how far I go doen the road of recovery, the ditch is still just as close.

Rule #3

The opposite of addiction is not sobriety, but community.

Rule #4

Yesterday's victory is no guarantee of tomorrow's success.

Rule #5

Recovery is about direction, not destination.

Rule #6

What I think today, I'll do tomorrow, and become the day after that.

Rule #7

Free cheese is always available in the mousetrap.

Rule #8

I am crippled by my addiction, but buried by my secrets.

Rule #9

I won't commit to a lifetime, just for a day.

Rule #10

God isn't going to use me despite my past, but because of it.

CPSIA information can be obtained
at www.ICGtesting.com
Printed in the USA
BVHW011620290520
580482BV00010B/306